P9-DFA-478

Bioethics
at the bedside

Generously donated by the
Joint Centre for Bioethics
Postgraduate Program

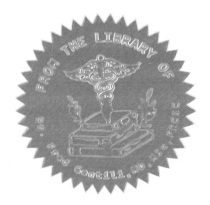

The CLINICAL BASICS Series

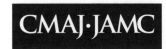

Bioethics
at the bedside

A CLINICIAN'S GUIDE

Edited by

Peter A. Singer

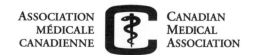

ASSOCIATION MÉDICALE CANADIENNE · CANADIAN MEDICAL ASSOCIATION

© 1999 Canadian Medical Association

All rights reserved. No part of this publication may be reproduced, stored in a retrieval system or transmitted in any form or by any means, electronic, mechanical, photocopying, recording or otherwise, without the prior written permission of the CMA or, in case of photocopying or other reprographic copying, a licence from CANCOPY (Canadian Copyright Licensing Agency), 6 Adelaide St. E, Suite 900, Toronto ON M5C 1H6 (800 893-5777).

Printed and bound in Canada

Canadian Cataloguing in Publication Data

Main entry under title:
    Bioethics at the bedside : a clinician's guide

Essays originally published in the Canadian Medical
    Association journal, Jul. 1996-Oct. 1998.
Includes bibliographical references.
ISBN 0-920169-31-7

    1. Medical ethics. 2. Bioethics. I. Singer, Peter A., 1960-
II. Canadian Medical Association.

R724.B56 1999   174'.2   C99-900058-6

All of the case histories in this book are fictitious. The opinions expressed are those of the authors and do not necessarily reflect the views of their supporting groups or employers. The information contained in this book is for reference and education only and is not intended to be a substitute for medical or legal advice. The CMA assumes no responsiblity for liability arising from any error in or omission from the book or from the use of any information contained in it.

Published by the Canadian Medical Association

Canadian Medical Association
1867 Alta Vista Drive
Ottawa ON K1G 3Y6
Telephone: 888 855-2555 or 613 731-8610 x2307 (Member Service Centre)
Fax: 613 236-8864
Email: cmamsc@cma.ca

Contents

Foreword

For many physicians the word "bioethics" might suggest a generally abstract and often thorny discipline pursued, quietly enough, in academic circles — except when groundbreaking cases complicated by legal wrangling and the collision of opposing values are debated in the mass media. Most of us watch from the sidelines, or think that we do. In reality, bioethics is a domain of questioning and awareness that physicians are engaged in every day of their working lives, in every encounter with patients and their families. This is bioethics at the bedside.

Most of the time the ethical underpinnings of our clinical practice are largely unconscious, deriving from personal background, societal context and the norms of professional conduct instilled during medical training. But sometimes it is worth pausing to reexamine the basis even of those judgements that seem routine. Occasionally, anomalous circumstances invite a closer look at first principles as we try to steer a course through an ethical dilemma. *Bioethics at the Bedside* provides a starting-point for these reflections.

Each chapter begins with a brief illustration of one or more ethical problems that physicians might encounter in everyday practice. The concepts at issue — ranging from informed consent and patient autonomy to research ethics and conflict of interest — are defined and their implications examined from the perspectives of ethical theory, law and policy. A practical approach to translating theory into practice is outlined and then demonstrated with a resolution of the sample cases. Each chapter covers the issues comprehensively and succinctly and can be read in sequence or used as a reference when specific problems arise.

This collection was originally published as a special series in the *Canadian Medical Association Journal* between July 1996 and October 1998. Former Editor-in-Chief Dr. Bruce Squires set the project in motion with the assistance of Dr. Patricia Huston, then Associate Editor-in-Chief. As series editor, Dr. Peter Singer, who is Sun Life Chair in Bioethics and Director of the University of Toronto Joint Centre for Bioethics, defined the scope of the series and identified contributors with the requisite interest and expertise in each area. We are grateful to Dr. Singer for his enthusiasm, energy and wise counsel during the entire project and to the authors for devoting much time and care to the writing and revision of each chapter. We are also indebted to the many reviewers who provided thoughtful critiques.

We hope that *Bioethics at the Bedside* will serve both physicians and their patients by providing a rational framework for decision-making in areas that are often beset by difficulty and doubt.

John Hoey, MD
Editor-in-Chief
Canadian Medical Association Journal

Preface

You probably faced an ethical issue in your practice today. Did you recognize it? Did you know how to address it? Did you have an organized framework? Did you know what to say to the patient and his or her family? Did you know what to do? Did you feel comfortable and confident in this aspect of your practice?

The paramount goal of teaching bioethics is to improve the quality of patient care by identifying, analysing and attempting to resolve the ethical problems that arise in the practice of clinical medicine.[1,2] Today, every medical school in Canada incorporates bioethics into its curriculum, and both the College of Family Physicians of Canada and the Royal College of Physicians and Surgeons of Canada require teaching of bioethics as a condition of accrediting residency programs. However, the extent to which education in bioethics informs and improves the clinician's work is unclear.

This book is intended to elucidate key concepts in bioethics and to help clinicians to integrate bioethical knowledge into daily practice. In educational terms, the goal is to support performance: what clinicians actually do.

Professional performance with respect to bioethical matters depends on many factors, including the clinician's values, beliefs, knowledge of ethical and legal constructs, ability to recognize and analyse ethical problems, and interpersonal and communications skills. Although this book cannot address every aspect of bioethics in medical practice, the authors hope that it will provide a helpful starting point for clinicians and complement bioethics educational initiatives such as those of the Royal College of Physicians and Surgeons of Canada, the College of Family Physicians of Canada and Canada's 16 medical schools.

This book has been written with the practising physician in mind. It should also be useful to educators teaching bioethics in medical schools, residency programs and continuing medical education. It may also be of use to nurses, social workers, physiotherapists, occupational therapists and other health care providers.

Topics were selected for their clinical relevance: consent, disclosure, capacity, voluntariness, substitute decision-making, advance care planning, truth telling, confidentiality, child health care ethics, maternal–fetal dilemmas, ethical issues in genetics, research ethics, euthanasia and assisted suicide, appropriate use of life-sustaining treatment, quality end-of-life care, resource allocation and conflict of interest.

Most chapters were written by a team of scholars in medicine, ethics and law. This interdisciplinary approach helps to ensure that concepts are described faithfully with respect to their empirical context in medicine and with an understanding of their theoretic roots in ethics and law.

Each chapter begins with one or more clinical cases highlighting the issue under discussion and ends with suggested approaches to these cases. The cases reflect the authors' experience and are not intended to refer to any particular patient. The cases are referred to sequentially by letter. In addition, each chapter answers 3 basic questions about the bioethical issue at hand: What is it? Why is it important? How should it be approached in practice?

Each chapter in this book was originally published as an article in the *Canadian Medical Association Journal* and has been individually peer reviewed. Reaction to the articles was positive. Practising physicians particularly liked their clinical focus and their brevity.

How will I know whether the series has succeeded? Ideally, I would measure the performance of Canada's 50 000 physicians in interactions with their 25 million patients. Obviously, this is not feasible. Therefore, I ask for your comments. Let me know what you think of the book (my email address is peter.singer@utoronto.ca). In particular, I would be interested in any impact the series might have on your practice. I look forward to hearing from you.

Peter A. Singer, MD, MPH
Sun Life Chair in Bioethics and
Director, University of Toronto Joint Centre for Bioethics
Associate Professor of Medicine, University of Toronto
Staff Physician, The Toronto Hospital
Medical Research Council of Canada Scientist

References

1. Siegler M. A legacy of Osler: teaching clinical ethics at the bedside. *JAMA* 1978;239:951-6.
2. Siegler M, Pellegrino ED, Singer PA. Clinical medical ethics. *J Clin Ethics* 1990;1:5-9.

Acknowledgements

Many people created this book. First, I am grateful to all the authors of articles in the *Canadian Medical Association Journal*'s Bioethics for Clinicians series, which became the chapters in this book. Second, I very much appreciate the efforts of the many anonymous peer reviewers who critiqued each article in the series and made it better. Third, I am grateful to Anne Marie Todkill and Gillian Pancirov of the Canadian Medical Association's Publishing Services, who provided excellent editorial assistance for the series and the book. Fourth, I am particularly appreciative of the support, encouragement and assistance of the *CMAJ* editors who nurtured the series and the book — John Hoey, Pat Huston and Bruce Squires. Fifth, I would like to thank all my colleagues at the University of Toronto Joint Centre for Bioethics for providing a wonderful professional environment in which this book could unfold. Sixth, I would like to thank the University of Toronto Joint Centre for Bioethics board members and their respective institutions for supporting this exciting partnership among the University of Toronto, Baycrest Centre for Geriatric Care, Centre for Addiction and Mental Health, The Hospital for Sick Children, Mount Sinai Hospital, Sunnybrook and Women's College Health Sciences Centre, The Toronto Hospital and the Toronto Rehabilitation Institute. Seventh, I thank the Medical Research Council of Canada, Health Canada and the Physicians Services Incorporated Foundation of Ontario for research support. Eighth, I would like to thank my mentors and friends, especially Arnie Aberman, Michael Baker, Allan Detsky, Alvan Feinstein, William Harvey, Herbert Ho Ping Kong, Fred Lowy, C. David Naylor, Eliot Phillipson, Mark Siegler and James G. Wright, for their support and encouragement. Most of all, I owe a debt of gratitude to my wife, Heather, and our children, David, Erin, and Rebecca for their love.

Peter A. Singer, MD, MPH

Contributors

Françoise Baylis, PhD
Associate Professor
Office of Bioethics Education
    and Research
Dalhousie University
Halifax, NS

Joseph M. Boyle, PhD*
Professor of Philosophy
University of Toronto
Toronto, Ont.

Michael M. Burgess, PhD
Centre for Applied Ethics
University of British Columbia
Vancouver, BC

Bernard M. Dickens, PhD, LLD*
Professor
Faculty of Law and
    Faculty of Medicine
University of Toronto
Toronto, Ont.

Mary Jane Dykeman, LLB
Health Law and Policy Consultant
Toronto, Ont.

Carl Elliott, MD, PhD
Center for Bioethics
University of Minnesota
Minneapolis, Minn.

Edward Etchells, MD, MSc*
Department of Medicine
The Toronto Hospital
University of Toronto
Toronto, Ont.

Elizabeth Flagler, MD
Associate Professor
Office of Medical Bioethics
University of Calgary
Calgary, Alta.

Kathleen C. Glass, LLB, DCL
Biomedical Ethics Unit
McGill University
Montreal, Que.

Glenn G. Griener, PhD
Associate Professor
University of Alberta
Edmonton, Alta.

Christine Harrison, PhD*
Director, Bioethics Department
The Hospital for Sick Children
Department of Pediatrics
University of Toronto
Toronto, Ont.

Philip C. Hébert, MD, PhD*
Department of Family and
    Community Medicine
Clinical Ethics Centre
Sunnybrook and Women's College
    Health Sciences Centre
University of Toronto
Toronto, Ont.

Barry Hoffmaster, PhD
Professor
Department of Philosophy and
    Department of Family Medicine
University of Western Ontario
London, Ont.

Nuala P. Kenny, MD
Professor, Department of Pediatrics
Director, Office of Bioethics
    Education and Research
Dalhousie University
Halifax, NS

Irwin Kleinman, MD*
Department of Psychiatry
Mount Sinai Hospital
University of Toronto
Toronto, Ont.

Bartha Maria Knoppers, LLD
Professor of Law
Centre de recherche en droit public
Université de Montréal
Montreal, Que.

Claude M. Laberge, MD, PhD
Professor
Centre Hospitalier
    de l'Université Laval
Sainte-Foy, Que.

James V. Lavery, MSc
Queen's University
Kingston General Hospital
Kingston, Ont.

Neil M. Lazar, MD*
Department of Medicine,
    Critical Care
The Toronto Hospital
University of Toronto
Toronto, Ont.

Trudo Lemmens, LicIur,
    LLM (Bioethics)*
Centre for Addiction and Mental
    Health
Department of Psychiatry and
Faculty of Law
University of Toronto
Toronto, Ont.

Neil MacDonald, CM, MD
Centre de bioéthique
Institut de recherches cliniques de
    Montréal
Professor of Oncology
McGill University
Montreal, Que.

Martin F. McKneally, MD, PhD*
Professor of Surgery
Department of Surgery
The Toronto Hospital
University of Toronto
Toronto, Ont.

Eric M. Meslin, PhD
Executive Director
National Bioethics Advisory
    Commission
Rockville, Md.

Gerald Robertson, LLB, LLM
Faculty of Law
University of Alberta
Edmonton, Alta.

Sanda Rodgers, LLB/BCL, LLM
Dean
Common Law Section
Faculty of Law
University of Ottawa
Ottawa, Ont.

Mary Rowell, MA, RN*
Bioethics Department
The Hospital for Sick Children
Department of Pediatrics
University of Toronto
Toronto, Ont.

David J. Roy, STL, PhL, DrTheol
Director, Centre for Bioethics
Clinical Research Institute
    of Montreal
Research Professor, Faculty
    of Medicine
Université de Montréal
Director, FRSQ Network for
    Research in Clinical Ethics
Montreal, Que.

Gilbert Sharpe, BA, LLB, LLM
Director, Legal Services Branch
Ontario Ministry of Health
Toronto, Ont.

Mona Sidarous, LLB, LLM
Université de Montréal
Montreal, Que.

Peter A. Singer, MD, MPH*
Sun Life Chair in Bioethics and
Director, University of Toronto
Joint Centre for Bioethics
Toronto, Ont.

Phil Walsh, BSc, LLB
Senior Editor
*Canadian Health Facilities Law
    Guide*
Toronto, Ont.

Charles Weijer, MD, PhD
Office for Bioethics Education and
    Research
Dalhousie University
Halifax, NS

John R. Williams, PhD
Director, Ethics
Canadian Medical Association
Ottawa, Ont.

Stephen Workman, MD, MSc
Associate Professor
Division of General Internal
    Medicine
Dalhousie University
Halifax, NS

*Member, University of Toronto
Joint Centre for Bioethics

Consent

Edward Etchells, MD, MSc; Gilbert Sharpe, BA, LLB, LLM;
Phil Walsh, BSc, LLB; John R. Williams, PhD; Peter A. Singer, MD, MPH

Mr. A is an 85-year-old man living at home with his wife, who has moderately severe Alzheimer's disease and for whom he provides daily care. He has an 8.5-cm abdominal aortic aneurysm. Three months ago he consulted a vascular surgeon, who recommended surgical repair of his aneurysm. However, another physician told Mr. A that he "would never survive the operation." Mr. A decided to "take his chances" and refused surgery, primarily because of his wish to provide uninterrupted care for his wife; however, he agreed to discuss the decision further with the surgeon at a future visit. Before such a visit takes place, however, Mr. A is taken to the emergency department after collapsing at home with abdominal pain. Physical examination reveals a systolic blood pressure of 50 mm Hg and a tender, pulsatile abdominal mass. Mr. A is moaning and barely conscious. The surgeon diagnoses a ruptured aortic aneurysm and believes that Mr. A will die without emergency surgery. No relatives can be reached for consultation.

Mr. B, a 69-year-old resident of a nursing home, has severe Alzheimer's disease. He is dependent on others to carry out all activities of daily living and is incontinent of urine and feces. He does not recognize his family members, and his speech is limited to moaning and crying. He has had fever, a cough producing green sputum and shortness of breath for 48 hours. He is transferred to hospital for treatment of suspected pneumonia. His wishes regarding treatment for pneumonia have not been documented. The nursing home has already notified Mr. B's wife, who is now driving to the hospital and will arrive in about 30 minutes.

What is consent?

"Consent" is the "autonomous authorization of a medical intervention . . . by individual patients."[1] Patients are entitled to make decisions about their medical care and have the right to be given all available information relevant to such decisions. Obtaining consent is not a discrete event; rather, it is a process that should occur throughout the relationship between clinician and patient.[2] Although the term "consent" implies acceptance of treatment, the concept of consent applies equally to refusal of treatment. Patients have the right to refuse treatment and to be given all available information relevant to the refusal.

Consent has 3 components: disclosure, capacity and voluntariness. "Disclosure" refers to the provision of relevant information by the clinician and its comprehension by the patient. "Capacity" refers to the patient's ability to understand the relevant information and to appreciate those consequences of his or her decision that might reasonably be foreseen. "Voluntariness" refers to the patient's right to come to a decision freely, without force, coercion or manipulation.

Consent may be explicit or implied.[3] Explicit consent can be given orally or in writing. Consent is implied when the patient indicates a willingness to undergo a certain procedure or treatment by his or her behaviour. For example, consent for venepuncture is implied by the action of rolling up one's sleeve and presenting one's arm. For treatments that entail risk or involve more than mild discomfort, explicit rather than implied consent should be obtained.

Signed consent forms document but cannot replace the consent process. There are no fixed rules as to when a signed consent form is required. Some hospitals require that a consent form be signed by the patient for surgical procedures but not for certain equally risky interventions. If a signed consent form is not required, and the treatment carries risk, clinicians should seriously consider writing a note in the patient's chart to document that the consent process has occurred.

In this chapter we will discuss the concept of patient consent and exceptions to the requirement to obtain consent. Subsequent chapters will provide a detailed discussion of disclosure, capacity and voluntariness, as well as requirements for patient consent to participation in medical research.

Why is consent important?

Ethics

The notion of consent is grounded in the ethical principles of patient autonomy and respect for persons. "Autonomy" refers to the patient's right to make free decisions about his or her health care. Respect for persons requires that health care professionals refrain from carrying out unwanted interventions and that they foster patients' control over their own lives.

Law

Obtaining the patient's consent to medical care is a legal requirement. Under common law, treating a patient without his or her consent constitutes battery,[4] whereas treating a patient on the basis of inadequately informed consent constitutes negligence.[5] Ontario's Health Care Consent Act (1996) defines the elements of consent, describes how capacity should be determined, allows patients to challenge a finding of incapacity and defines who may give consent on behalf of the patient.[6] British Columbia[7] and Prince Edward Island[8] are in the process of enacting similar legislation.

Policy

The requirement to obtain patient consent is affirmed by professional organizations such as the Royal College of Physicians and Surgeons of Canada, the Canadian Council on Hospital Accreditation and the Canadian Medical Association (CMA). For example, the CMA's policy summary on informed decision-making states: "Obtaining valid consent before carrying out medical, therapeutic and diagnostic procedures has long been recognized as an elementary step in fulfilling the doctor's obligations to the patient."[9]

Empirical studies

Several meta-analyses and reviews have suggested that the process of obtaining consent can be an important component of a successful physician–patient relationship. One review found that effective physician–patient communication improved emotional health, symptom resolution, level of function, results of physiologic measures and pain control.[10] A meta-analysis showed that providing information about what the patient would feel and what would be done in the course of stressful and painful medical procedures consistently reduced negative feelings, pain and distress.[11] Another demonstrated that information-giving by physicians was associated with small to moderate increases in patient satisfaction and compliance with treatment.[12]

How should I approach the consent process in practice?

Problem-solving and decision-making

Clinicians often struggle with the question of how to apply the ethical and legal concept of consent in their daily practice. It is helpful to distinguish the process of problem-solving from that of decision-making.[13] Problem-solving involves identifying the patient's presenting problem and developing a list of treatment options. Most patients expect the physician to assume the role of problem solver.[14,15] Decision-making involves choosing from the treatment options. Several studies have shown that patients' desire for decision-making responsibility is variable.[16-23] Even patients who actively seek information do not necessarily wish to make the decision about which treatment option to follow.[24,25] Some, particularly those who are elderly or acutely ill, are predisposed to follow the physician's recommendation.[26-28]

Obtaining valid consent requires that patients participate in problem-solving as much as they wish. Patients should be free to ask questions and receive answers about treatment options not discussed by the clinician. The consent process also requires that patients actively participate in decision-making and authorize the decision. Even if the patient is predisposed to follow the clinician's recommendation, the clinician should actively engage the patient in the consent process.

Exceptions

Common law recognizes that the emergency treatment of incapable persons is an exception to the requirement for consent. In common law, an emergency exists when immediate treatment is required to save the life or preserve the health of the patient.[29] The rationale for this exception is that a reasonable person would consent to the treatment and that a delay in treatment would lead to death or serious harm. In some provinces an emergency may be defined differently in statutory law than in common law, and so clinicians should be aware of the legislation in their own province. In Ontario statutory law, for example, an emergency exists if a person is apparently experiencing severe suffering or is at risk, if the treatment is not administered promptly, of sustaining serious bodily harm.[30]

The emergency exception to the requirement to obtain consent has important limitations. Clinicians should not administer emergency treatment without consent if they have reason to believe that the patient would refuse such treatment if he or she were capable. For example, in *Malette* v. *Shulman*[4] the physician gave a blood transfusion to a patient who, because of shock and severe facial injuries, was unconscious. The patient carried a signed card indicating that she was a Jehovah's Witness who did not want to receive blood transfusions under any circumstances. Despite this information, blood transfusions were given. Although the transfusions probably saved the patient's life, the court found the clinician liable for battery, holding that the written instructions were "clear, precise and unequivocal"[31] and that the clinician was bound by them unless he had good reason to believe that they did not truly represent the patient's wishes.[31]

A patient's incapacity does not exempt the physician from the requirement to obtain consent. If a patient is mentally incapable of making medical decisions, the clinician must obtain consent from a substitute. Assessing capacity and obtaining substitute consent will be discussed in detail in later chapters.

The statutory law of some provinces permits nonconsensual treatment in specific circumstances, such as the involuntary admission of psychiatric patients and the treatment of irresponsible patients with communicable disease.

There are other potential exceptions to the requirement to obtain consent. "Therapeutic privilege" refers to the physician's withholding of certain information in the consent process in the belief that disclosure of this information would harm or cause suffering to the patient.[30] "Waiver" refers to a patient's voluntary request to forgo one or more elements of disclosure. Therapeutic privilege and waiver will be discussed in chapter 2.

Mr. A' s physician must decide whether to perform surgical repair of the aneurysm. Mr. A. is now an incapable person in a medical emergency, and no substitute decision-maker is available. In such a circumstance the surgeon may proceed without the patient's consent unless a clear wish to the contrary has been expressed earlier. Should the surgeon proceed, given that Mr. A had previously refused elective repair of the aneurysm? Mr. A's refusal of elective surgery was based on his wish to continue caring for his wife. Therefore, Mr. A would likely want to undergo emergency surgery, because it would give him the best chance of continuing to care for his wife. Therefore, the surgeon may proceed without the patient's consent. If Mr. A had previously considered and refused emergency surgery, the surgeon would not be entitled to proceed.

Mr. B is obviously incapable of consenting to treatment of his pneumonia, and so the physician should obtain consent from Mr. B's wife. However, the clinician could administer emergency treatment such as oxygen and intravenous antibiotic therapy until Mr. B's wife arrives.

References

1. Beauchamp TL, Faden RR. Informed consent: II. Meaning and elements of informed consent. In: Reich WT, editor. *Encyclopedia of bioethics.* rev ed. vol 3. New York: Simon & Schuster Macmillan; 1995. p. 1240.
2. Lidz CW, Appelbaum PS, Meisel A. Two models of implementing informed consent. *Arch Intern Med* 1988;148:1385-9.
3. Canadian Medical Protective Association. *Consent. A guide for Canadian physicians.* Ottawa: The Association; 1989. p. 7.

4. *Malette* v. *Shulman* (1990), 67 DLR (4th) 321 at 338 (Ont CA).
5. *Reibl* v. *Hughes*, [1980] 2 SCR 880.
6. *Health Care Consent Act*, SO 1996, c 2.
7. *Health Care and Care Facility Act*, SBC 1993, c 48.
8. *Consent to Treatment and Health Care Directives Act*, SPEI 1996, c 10.
9. Informed decision-making [policy summary]. *CMAJ* 1986;135:1208A.
10. Stewart MA. Effective physician–patient communication and health outcomes: a review. *CMAJ* 1995;152:1423-33.
11. Suls J, Wan CK. Effects of sensory and procedural information on coping with stressful medical procedures and pain: a meta analysis. *J Consult Clin Psychol* 1989;57:372-9.
12. Hall JA, Roter DL, Katz NR. Meta-analysis of correlates of provider behavior in medical encounters. *Med Care* 1988;26:657-75.
13. Deber RB. Physicians in health care management: 8. The patient–physician partnership: decision making, problem solving and the desire to participate. *CMAJ* 1994;151:423-7.
14. Kraetschmer N. Preferences of patients undergoing angiograms for participation in treatment decisions: coping style and the problem solving–decision-making scale [master's thesis]. Toronto: University of Toronto; 1994.
15. Siminoff LA, Fetting JH. Factors affecting treatment decisions for a life-threatening illness: the case of medical treatment of breast cancer. *Soc Sci Med* 1991;32:813-8.
16. Cassileth BR, Zupkis RV, Sutton-Smith K, March V. Information and participation preferences among cancer patients. *Ann Intern Med* 1980;92:832-6.
17. Ende J, Kazis L, Ash A, Moskowitz MA. Measuring patients' desire for autonomy: decision making and information-seeking preferences among medical patients. *J Gen Intern Med* 1989;4:23-30.
18. Larsson US, Svardsudd K, Wedel H, Saljo R. Patient involvement in decision-making in surgical and orthopaedic practice: the Project Perioperative Risk. *Soc Sci Med* 1989;28:829-35.
19. Ende J, Kazis L, Moskowitz MA. Preferences for autonomy when patients are physicians. *J Gen Intern Med* 1990;5:506-9.
20. Lerman CE, Brody DS, Caputo GC, Smith DG, Lazaro CG, Wolfson HG. Patients' Perceived Involvement in Care Scale: relationship to attitudes about illness and medical care. *J Gen Intern Med* 1990;5:29-33.
21. Mark JS, Spiro H. Informed consent for colonoscopy. *Arch Intern Med* 1990;150:777-80.
22. Llewellyn-Thomas HA, McGreal MJ, Thiel EC, Fine S, Erlichman C. Patients' willingness to enter clinical trials: measuring the association with perceived benefit and preference for decision participation. *Soc Sci Med* 1991;32:35-42.
23. Waterworth S, Luker KA. Reluctant collaborators: Do patients want to be involved in decisions concerning care? *J Adv Nurs* 1990;15:971-6.
24. Sutherland HJ, Llewellyn-Thomas HA, Lockwood GA, Tritchler DL, Till JE. Cancer patients: their desire for information and participation in treatment decisions. *J R Soc Med* 1989;82:260-3.
25. Blanchard CG, Labrecque MS, Ruckdeschel JC, Blanchard EB. Information and decision-making preferences of hospitalized adult cancer patients. *Soc Sci Med* 1988;27:1139-45.
26. Emanuel EJ, Emanuel LL. Four models of the physician–patient relationship. *JAMA* 1992;267:2221-6.
27. Strull WM, Lo B, Charles G. Do patients want to participate in medical decision making? *JAMA* 1984;252:2990-4.

28. Beisecker AE, Beisecker TD. Patient information-seeking behaviors when communicating with doctors. *Med Care* 1990;28:19-28.
29. *Malette* v. *Shulman* (1990), 67 DLR (4th) 321 at 328 (Ont CA).
30. *Health Care Consent Act*, SO 1996, c 2, s 25.
31. *Malette* v. *Shulman* (1990), 67 DLR (4th) 321 at 337 (Ont CA).

Acknowledgement: Ms. Sharon Smith for careful preparation of the manuscript.

2

Disclosure

Edward Etchells, MD, MSc; Gilbert Sharpe, BA, LLB, LLM;
Michael M. Burgess, PhD; Peter A. Singer, MD, MPH

Mr. C is 61 years old and works as a supervisor at a car assembly plant. He lives at home with his wife. He has been in good health, although he smokes a pack of cigarettes a day. At a routine checkup his physician notes a loud bruit at the left carotid artery. Mr. C, who is right handed, has never had a transient ischemic attack or stroke. Duplex Doppler ultrasonography reveals significant stenosis of the left internal carotid artery; cerebral angiography reveals the degree of the stenosis to be 95%. Carotid endarterectomy is recommended; Mr. C discusses this proposal with the consultant vascular surgeon.

Mrs. D is 75 years old and lives at home with her husband. She has a remote history of gastric ulcers and has mild renal insufficiency as a consequence of hypertension. She visits her family physician because of acute worsening of chronic arthritis in her right shoulder. She is having trouble lifting and carrying objects. Her family physician is considering treating Mrs. D with a nonsteroidal anti-inflammatory drug (NSAID).

Mrs. E is 80 years old and lives alone in an apartment. She is fully independent and has never had a serious illness. She prefers not to see doctors. She is admitted to hospital after falling on the stairs and suffering a fracture of the femoral neck. A consultant in internal medicine diagnoses critical aortic stenosis; this is confirmed by echocardiography. The anesthetist visits Mrs. E to discuss the proposed surgery and anesthesia. When he says that serious risks are associated with the surgery, Mrs. E says she does not want to know about them. She wants her hip fixed because she simply cannot live with reduced mobility. The anesthetist feels that he has a duty to disclose the risks of anesthesia.

Ms. F is 28 years old. She was admitted to hospital 6 weeks ago with an exacerbation of poorly controlled asthma. The hospital internist prescribed long-term oral corticosteroid therapy. Ms. F is now taking prednisone (20 mg/d) and has noticed weight gain and mood disturbance. She thinks that she should stop taking the medication. Her family physician has recently read about a case of avascular necrosis of the femoral head associated with prednisone therapy, but he believes that prednisone therapy is important to control Ms. F's asthma. He wonders whether the risk of avascular necrosis should not be disclosed, lest this information cause Ms. F to stop taking prednisone.

What is disclosure?

"Disclosure," in the context of patient consent, refers to both the provision of relevant information by the clinician and its comprehension by the patient. Both elements are necessary for valid consent.

Why is disclosure important?

Ethics

In keeping with the ethical principles of patient autonomy and respect for persons, disclosure promotes patients' informed and reflective participation in health care decisions. Disclosure also promotes a continuing and trusting relationship between patient and physician.[1,2]

Law
Elements of disclosure

The necessary elements of disclosure as identified in Canadian statutory[3,4] and common[5] law are as follows: a description of the treatment and its expected effects (e.g., duration of hospital stay, expected time to recovery, restrictions on daily activities, scars); information about relevant alternative options and their expected benefits and relevant risks; and an explanation of the consequences of declining or delaying treatment. The patient must be given an opportunity to ask questions, and the clinician must respond to questions or requests for further information.

Scope of disclosure

In Canada, the prevailing standard of disclosure is that of the "reasonable person."[3-5] This is an objective standard that requires the clinician to disclose information that a reasonable person in the patient's position would need in order to make an informed decision. The concept of "a reasonable person in the patient's position" may be understood by an example regarding disclosure of risks. Mr. C is considering carotid endarterectomy for asymptomatic stenosis of the carotid artery. Carotid endarterectomy has a known risk of immediate death or stroke. These risks must be disclosed, because a risk of death, paralysis or permanent loss of a body function would be relevant (or "material") to a reasonable person. However, Mr. C is within 6 months of obtaining full pension benefits at work. A reasonable person in Mr. C's financial position would also need to know that the risk of having a stroke in the next 6 months would be higher with endarterectomy than with medical treatment.[6] In Canada, the reasonable-person standard for disclosure was established by the Supreme Court of Canada in the case of *Reibl* v. *Hughes*,[5] upon which the case of Mr. C is based.

Waiver

"Waiver" refers to a patient's voluntary request to forgo one or more elements of disclosure. For example, a patient may not wish to know about a serious prognosis (e.g., cancer) or about the risks of treatment. Because Canadian legislation and common law do not directly address the issue of waiver, clinicians should proceed cautiously when a patient appears to be requesting a waiver.

Therapeutic privilege

"Therapeutic privilege" refers to the withholding of information by the clinician during the consent process in the belief that disclosure of this information would lead to the harm or suffering of the patient.[7]

The legal status of therapeutic privilege in Canada is uncertain. The case of *Meyer Estate* v. *Rogers*[8] involved a 37-year-old woman who died after intravenous injection of a contrast medium for a routine radiologic procedure. The radiologist claimed therapeutic privilege as a defence against the allegation that he failed to warn the patient of the risks of intravenous dye injection. The court rejected the defence on the grounds that therapeutic privilege was not applicable.[8] The judge concluded that "the Supreme Court of Canada has not . . . adopted or even approved the therapeutic privilege exception in Canada."[9]

The need for sensitivity to cultural norms may potentially support the exercise of therapeutic privilege. In some cultures therapeutic privilege is widely invoked, and it is unclear whether patients from these cultures should always be subjected to Western standards of consent.[10] However, given the legal status of therapeutic privilege in Canada, clinicians should avoid invoking therapeutic privilege. It is better for the clinician to offer information and allow the patient to refuse or accept further disclosure.

Policy

Disclosure is an essential component of valid consent, and obtaining valid consent is a policy of the CMA[11] and other professional bodies.

Empirical studies

The results of empirical studies of disclosure suggest that patients' desire for information closely agrees with the legal standard for disclosure. In one study more than 80% of a sample of surgical patients wanted to know about the nature of their illness, the reason for the surgery, the nature of the operation, the expected duration of their stay in hospital, the chances of a successful result, the expected time to return to normal daily activities and any special precautions they would need to take after surgery.[12] Similar observations have been made with regard to patients' desire for information about anesthesia.[13–15]

Studies have indicated that 6% to 18% of patients prefer not to know about the risks of treatment.[12,13,16] However, this research evaluated patients who had already decided to proceed with surgery or had already undergone successful surgery and did not address the question of what they wanted to know about risks in order to consent to surgery.

Most studies in this area have found that routine verbal disclosure is not completely effective,[17–25] whereas written[26–30] or combined written and verbal disclosure[31–34] can improve patients' knowledge. Other aids to disclosure, such as bedside decision instruments[35] and interactive videodiscs,[36] are promising but require further evaluation.

How should I approach disclosure in practice?

Disclosure should be viewed as a process rather than as a discrete event. Several encounters between the clinician and patient may be needed before disclosure can be considered complete. For example, Ms. F and her clinician may need to discuss prednisone therapy on a number of occasions to ensure proper disclosure of benefits and risks. If a therapy is given over a prolonged period the disclosure process should continue. For example, if new information relevant to a patient's drug therapy becomes available it should be disclosed.

Effective communication is critical to the disclosure process. If the clinician fosters good communication the patient will be encouraged to provide personal information and express his or her values, goals and fears. A full discussion of effective physician–patient communication is beyond the scope of this chapter, but several relevant reviews are available.[37–41]

During the consent process clinicians should routinely address each element of disclosure, giving information about each of the areas described earlier (see "Elements of disclosure"). The goal is to disclose any information that a reasonable person in the patient's circumstances would want to know. Depending on the treatment in question, clinicians may need to consider how it, and other options, could affect the patient's employment, finances, family life and other personal concerns.

Disclosure should also take account of the patient's cultural and religious beliefs. For example, in some cultures a family-centred model of decision-making is favoured over one centred on the individual.[42] The clinician can encourage patients in such a situation to involve family members in the consent process. Although cultural sensitivity is a complex issue beyond the scope of this chapter, several reviews are helpful.[10,43,44]

Throughout each disclosure session the clinician should invite questions. Encouraging patients to restate information in their own words is one way to ensure that information has been understood. The clinician should document each discussion, noting the patient's questions and how these were answered. Special cultural or religious considerations are particularly important to document.

The surgeon asks Mr. C if he has any worries or concerns about the proposed surgery and learns that Mr. C is due for full pension benefits in 6 months. The surgeon discloses that the risk of stroke within 6 months is higher with surgery than with medical treatment. Subsequently, the surgeon and Mr. C agree to continue acetylsalicylic acid therapy, to arrange for Mr. C's enrolment in a smoking cessation program and to re-evaluate the treatment decision in 6 months. The surgeon's note includes the reasons for the decision and a reminder of why Mr. C will return in 6 months.

Mrs. D has no questions about the "arthritis pill" because she trusts her physician, whom she has known for many years. The physician initiates a discussion of the risks — in particular, gastrointestinal bleeding and renal insufficiency. Mrs. D appears concerned, and the clinician invites her to discuss this concern. Mrs. D explains that the shoulder pain must be relieved so that she can care for her young granddaughter, who will be visiting next month. The physician mentions that acetaminophen may also be effective and has a lower risk of side effects. Although pain relief is a high priority, Mrs. D would prefer to avoid side effects, particularly because she was once admitted to hospital because of her gastric ulcer. She agrees to try acetaminophen therapy for 2 weeks and if there is no effect to then try the NSAID. The physician makes a note of their discussion and arranges a follow-up appointment for 2 weeks hence.

Mrs. E has asked the anesthetist not to disclose further the risks associated with hip surgery. She says that her goal is to be able to walk and that further suffering from pain and immobility is not acceptable to her. She tells the anesthetist that any further discussion of risks will not change her mind but might upset her. The anesthetist respects Mrs. E's request but tells her that she can change her mind regarding the discussion of risks at any time. He also asks her if there are family members whom Mrs. E would like to involve in the decision-making process. Mrs. E wants her daughters to participate in the decision, and so the proposed surgery and its possible risks are disclosed to them. The entire discussion is documented, including Mrs. E's reasons for waiving further disclosure of the risks of surgery. Mrs. E undergoes uncomplicated repair of her hip fracture and returns home to live independently.

Ms. F should be informed of the risk of avascular necrosis of the femoral head. The clinician should not use therapeutic privilege to justify withholding this information.

References

1. President's Commission for the Study of Ethical Problems in Medicine and Biomedical and Behavioural Research, editor. *Making health care decisions, volume one: report.* Washington: The Commission; 1982.
2. Burgess MM. Informed consent: a medical ethicist's perspective. *Ann R Coll Physicians Surg Can* 1985;18:491-3.
3. *Health Care and Care Facility Act*, SBC 1993, c 48, s 6.
4. *Health Care Consent Act*, SO 1996, c 2, s 11.
5. *Reibl* v. *Hughes*, [1980] 2 SCR 880.
6. Executive Committee for the Asymptomatic Carotid Atherosclerosis Study. Endarterectomy for asymptomatic carotid artery stenosis. *JAMA* 1995;273:1421-8.
7. Meisel A, Roth LH, Lidz CW. Toward a model of the legal doctrine of informed consent. *Am J Psychiatry* 1977;134:285-9.
8. *Meyer Estate* v. *Rogers* (1991), 2 OR (3d) 356 (Gen Div).
9. *Meyer Estate* v. *Rogers* (1991), 2 OR (3d) 356 at 364 (Gen Div), note 4.
10. Williams JR. Ethics in cross-cultural health. In: Masi R, McLeod K, Mensah L, editors. *Health and culture: exploring the relationships. vol. 1: policy, practices, and education.* Oakville (ON): Mosaic Press; 1993. p. 255-70.
11. Canadian Medical Association. Informed decision-making [policy summary]. *CMAJ* 1986;135:1208A.
12. Dawes PJD, Davison P. Informed consent: What do patients want to know? *J R Soc Med* 1994;87:149-52.
13. Farnill D, Inglis S. Patients' desire for information about anaesthesia: Australian attitudes. *Anaesthesia* 1993;48:162-4.
14. Shevde K, Panagopoulos G. A survey of 800 patients' knowledge, attitudes, and concerns regarding anesthesia. *Anesth Analg* 1991;73:190-8.
15. Lonsdale M, Hutchison GL. Patients' desire for information about anaesthesia. *Anaesthesia* 1991;46:410-2.
16. Bunker TD. An information leaflet for surgical patients. *Ann R Coll Surg Engl* 1983;65:242-3.
17. Dunkelman H. Patients' knowledge of their condition and treatment: how it might be improved. *BMJ* 1979;2:311-4.

18. Cassileth BR, Zupkis RV, Sutton-Smith K, March V. Informed consent: Why are its goals imperfectly realized? *N Engl J Med* 1980;302:896-900.
19. Layton SA. Informed consent in oral and maxillofacial surgery: a study of its efficacy. *Br J Oral Maxillofac Surg* 1992;30:319-22.
20. Byrne DJ, Napier A, Cuschieri A. How informed is signed consent? *BMJ* 1988;296:839-40.
21. Muss HB, White DR, Michielutte R, Richards F 2d, Cooper MR, Williams S, et al. Written informed consent in patients with breast cancer. *Cancer* 1979;43:1549-56.
22. Sutherland HJ, Lockwood G, Till JE. Are we getting informed consent from patients with cancer? *J R Soc Med* 1990;83:439-43.
23. Robinson G, Merav A. Informed consent: recall by patients tested postoperatively. *Ann Thorac Surg* 1976;22:209-12.
24. Wade TC. Patients may not recall disclosure of risk of death: implications for informed consent. *Med Sci Law* 1990;30:259-62.
25. Lyunoe N, Sandlund M, Dahlqvist G, Jacobsson L. Informed consent: study of quality of information given to participants in a clinical trial. *BMJ* 1991;303:610-3.
26. Gibbs S, Waters WE, George CF. Communicating information to patients about medicine. *J R Soc Med* 1990;83:292-7.
27. Hopper KD, Tyler HN. Informed consent for intravascular administration of contrast material: How much is enough? *Radiology* 1989;171:509-14.
28. Askew G, Pearson KW, Cryer D. Informed consent: Can we educate patients? *J R Coll Surg Edinb* 1990;35:308-10.
29. Gates RA, Weaver MJ, Gates RH. Patient acceptance of an information sheet about cardiopulmonary resuscitation options. *J Gen Intern Med* 1993;8:679-82.
30. Tymchuk AJ, Ouslander JG, Rahbar B, Fitten J. Medical decision-making among elderly people in long-term care. *Gerontologist* 1988;28:59-63.
31. Dawes PJD, O'Keefe L, Adcock S. Informed consent: the assessment of two structured interview approaches compared to the current approach. *J Laryngol Otol* 1992;106:420-4.
32. Kleinman I, Schachter D, Jeffries J, Goldhamer P. Effectiveness of two methods for informing schizophrenic patients about neuroleptic medication. *Hosp Community Psychiatry* 1993;44:1189-91.
33. Layton S, Korsen J. Informed consent in oral and maxillofacial surgery: a study of the value of written warnings. *Br J Oral Maxillofac Surg* 1994;32:34-6.
34. Simes RJ, Tattersall MHN, Coates AS, Raghaven D, Solomon HJ. Randomised comparison of procedures for obtaining informed consent in clinical trials of treatment for cancer. *BMJ* 1986;293:1065-8.
35. Levine MN, Gafnie A, Markham B, MacFarlane D. A bedside decision instrument to elicit a patient's preference concerning adjuvant chemotherapy for breast cancer. *Ann Intern Med* 1992;117:53-8.
36. Ader DN, Seibring AR, Bhaskar P, Melamed BG. Information seeking and interactive videodisc preparation for third molar extraction. *J Oral Maxillofac Surg* 1992;50:27-31.
37. Beckman HB, Frankel RM. The effect of physician behavior on the collection of data. *Ann Intern Med* 1984;101:692-6.
38. Waitzkin H. Doctor–patient communication: clinical implications of social scientific research. *JAMA* 1984;252:2441-6.
39. Epstein AM, Taylor WC, Seage GR. Effects of patients' socioeconomic status and physicians' training and practice on patient–doctor communication. *Am J Med* 1985;78:101-6.

40. Matthews DA, Feinstein AR. A review of systems for the personal aspects of patient care. *Am J Med Sci* 1988;295:159-71.
41. Quill TE. Recognizing and adjusting to barriers in doctor–patient communication. *Ann Intern Med* 1989;111:51-7.
42. Blackhall LJ, Murphy ST, Frank G, Michel V, Azen S. Ethnicity and attitudes toward patient autonomy. *JAMA* 1995;274:820-5.
43. Jecker NS, Carrese JA, Pearlman RA. Caring for patients in cross-cultural settings. *Hastings Cent Rep* 1995;25(1):6-14.
44. Espino DV, editor. Ethnogeriatrics [special issue]. *Clin Geriatr Med* 1995;11(1).

3

Capacity

Edward Etchells, MD, MSc; Gilbert Sharpe, BA, LLB, LLM;
Carl Elliott, MD, PhD; Peter A. Singer, MD, MPH

Mr. G is 42 years old and is receiving neuroleptic therapy for chronic schizophrenia. Although he is unemployed he functions independently in the community. Because he believes that his neighbours break into his house and steal his money when he is out, he rarely leaves his apartment. He calls his family physician because of a sore throat. The physician makes a house call and obtains a throat swab, which reveals a *Streptococcus pyogenes* infection. The physician recommends antibiotic therapy.

Mr. H is a 65-year-old man admitted to hospital because of acute imbalance and clumsiness in the left arm. Atrial fibrillation and infarction of the left cerebellar hemisphere are diagnosed. His clinician recommends warfarin therapy, but Mr. H repeatedly refuses.

Mrs. I is a 79-year-old woman with noninsulin-dependent diabetes mellitus who is admitted to hospital with gangrene of the first and second toes of her right foot. She lives alone and does not like doctors. She receives intravenous antibiotic therapy for 1 week without response. Her clinicians recommend amputation of the affected toes, but she says, "I don't know what you will do with them after you cut them off."

Mr. J is 74 years old and has severe Parkinson's disease. He is admitted to hospital with psychosis caused by bromocriptine therapy. His clinician wishes to start treatment with clozapine, an antipsychotic drug with minimal extrapyramidal side effects but potentially severe hematologic side effects. When the clinician attempts to obtain consent Mr. J is unable to respond to any questions.

What is capacity?

"Capacity," or "decision-making capacity," is the ability to understand information relevant to a decision and to appreciate the reasonably foreseeable consequences of a decision or lack of decision. Capacity is specific to particular decisions: a person may be capable with respect to deciding about a place of residence, for example, but incapable with respect to deciding about a treatment. Capacity can change over time. For example, a person may be temporarily incapable because of delirium but subsequently recover his or her capacity.

Why is capacity important?

Ethics

The ethical principles of patient autonomy and respect for persons require that capable people be allowed to make their own informed decisions. However, the ethical principle of physician beneficence requires that incapable people be protected from making decisions that are harmful or that they would not make if they were capable.

Law

In law, capable patients are entitled to make their own informed decisions. If a patient is incapable the physician must obtain consent from a designated substitute decision-maker. In common law and under some legislation patients are presumed capable. If it is unreasonable to presume capacity, then a capacity assessment should be undertaken.

In Canadian common law there is no age below which a person is not presumed capable. A minor can give consent if he or she is able to understand the information about a treatment and to appreciate the risks and likely consequences of the treatment.[1] Some provinces have legislation that establishes the age of consent to treatment (Table 1); clinicians should familiarize themselves with the legislative requirements in their own province.

Policy

Capacity is an essential component of valid consent, and obtaining valid consent is a policy of the CMA[7] and other professional bodies.

How should I approach capacity in practice?

A clinician develops a general impression of a patient's capacity during the clinical encounter. In most cases the clinician has little reason to question the patient's capacity and focuses on other aspects of the consent process.

Table 1: Age of consent for medical treatment in Canada	
Prince Edward Island	A person must be at least 18 years of age or married to consent to surgery in a public hospital.[2]
New Brunswick	The age of consent for medical treatment is 16 years. A younger person may consent if, in the opinion of the attending physician or dentist and a second physician or dentist, he or she is capable of understanding the nature and consequences of treatment, and the treatment is in the person's best interests with respect to continued health and well-being.[3]
Quebec	The age of consent is 14 years if the treatment is required because of the patient's state of health. For a child under 14 years of age parental consent must be obtained unless a judge orders otherwise or if the child's life is in danger.[4]
Saskatchewan	A person must be at least 18 years of age or married to consent to surgery in a public hospital.[5]
British Columbia	A person who has reached the age of 16 years can consent to treatment if the health care provider has made a reasonable attempt to obtain consent from the person with parental authority and a written opinion is obtained from a second physician or dentist that the treatment is in the person's best interests with respect to continued health and well-being.[6]
Other provinces	The remaining provinces have no legislation that establishes an age of consent to treatment. In common law there is no age of consent. A minor can consent if he or she is capable of understanding the information about a treatment and of appreciating the risks and likely consequences of treatment.[1]

However, some patients, such as those who are comatose or who have severe dementia, are obviously incapable. In such cases the clinical assessment of capacity is straightforward, and substitute consent is required. (Substitute decision-making is discussed in chapter 5.)

In some situations clinicians may be unsure about a patient's capacity. The patient may have a neurologic or psychiatric disease or may be behaving in a way that indicates lack of understanding. Although refusal of recommended treatment may cause a clinician to *question* a person's capacity,[8] refusal of treatment should not be considered evidence of incapacity.[9] Most refusals are caused by factors other than incapacity.[10]

When a clinician is unsure about a patient's capacity an assessment is needed. The initial objective of assessment is to screen for incapacity.

Patients who appear to be incapable after the screening assessment generally require further assessment. Clinicians may use 3 different measures of capacity: cognitive function testing, general impressions of capacity and specific capacity assessments.

Cognitive function tests such as the Mini Mental State Examination[11] are reliable, easy to administer and familiar to clinicians in a wide variety of settings. However, although cognition and capacity are related, they are not identical.[12-15] Most measures of cognitive status do not evaluate several cognitive functions, such as judgement and reasoning, that are relevant to capacity.[16] A person may have a perfect cognitive test score but still be incapable by virtue of delusions that directly affect the treatment decision. Another limitation of cognitive status tests is that cut-off scores for identifying incapacity have not been established.

Gaining a general impression of a patient's capacity is a simple and quick method of assessment but can be unreliable,[17] inaccurate[13,14] and easily biased.[18]

In a specific capacity assessment the clinician discloses information relevant to the treatment decision and then evaluates the person's ability to understand this information and to appreciate the consequences of his or her decision. The Aid to Capacity Evaluation is a decisional aid to assist clinicians in carrying out specific capacity assessments.[19] It prompts clinicians to probe 7 relevant areas (Table 2), provides sample questions for the evaluation of each area and gives suggestions for scoring. Other decisional aids have been developed to assist with the assessment of the

Table 2: Relevant areas of patient capacity specified in the Aid to Capacity Evaluation[19]
Ability to understand the medical problem
Ability to understand the proposed treatment
Ability to understand the alternatives (if any) to the proposed treatment
Ability to understand the option of refusing treatment or of it being withheld or withdrawn
Ability to appreciate the reasonably foreseeable consequences of accepting the proposed treatment
Ability to appreciate the reasonably forseeable consequences of refusing the proposed treatment
Ability to make a decision that is not substantially based on delusions or depression

patient's capacity to complete an advance directive,[20] to consent to treatment[21-26] and to assist with the simultaneous assessment of several types of capacity.[27]

Specific capacity assessments have several strengths. First, they directly assess the patient's actual functioning while he or she is making a decision, which is exactly what the legal definition of capacity requires. Second, they are clinically feasible and quick: the median time for Aid to Capacity Evaluation is 12 minutes.[19] Finally, specific capacity assessments are flexible and can easily be adapted to various clinical circumstances.

However, specific capacity assessments have certain drawbacks. First, they are only as good as the accompanying disclosure. If the clinician does not disclose information effectively, the capacity assessment will be inaccurate. Therefore, excellent communication skills are critical to accurate assessment. In practice the process of disclosure should continue throughout the capacity assessment. For example, if a patient does not initially appreciate that he or she may be able to walk after a below-knee amputation, then this information should be redisclosed. Then the clinician can re-evaluate whether this consequence of below-knee amputation has been understood.

A second problem with specific capacity assessments relates to the evaluation of a patient's reasons for a decision. The goal is to ensure that the decision is not substantially based on a delusion and is not the result of depression. However, some "delusions" may represent personal, religious or cultural values that are not appreciated by the clinician. Similarly, it is difficult to determine whether a decision is substantially affected by the cognitive features of depression, such as hopelessness and feelings of worthlessness, guilt and persecution.[28,29]

A third problem is that a patient's capacity may fluctuate. If a person appears to be incapable the clinician should determine whether any reversible factors such as delirium or a drug reaction are at work. If such factors are identified the clinician should attempt to eliminate or minimize them and then repeat the assessment. There may also be factors that prevent a person from communicating effectively with the clinician, such as a language barrier or speech disturbance. Such factors must be addressed to ensure accurate capacity assessment.

Finally, clinicians may find it difficult to perform unbiased capacity assessments, particularly when the patient's choice goes against their recommendations. It is important to remember that agreement or disagreement with the patient's decision is not at issue; the purpose of capacity assessment is to evaluate the person's ability to understand relevant information and to appreciate the consequences of a decision.

If the result of screening indicates that a patient may be incapable, further expert assessment is generally recommended, particularly if the clinician is unsure about the assessment or if the person challenges the finding of incapacity. Expert assessments can be conducted by individual practitioners (e.g., psychiatrists and psychologists), hospital ethics committees or legal review boards. If a finding of incapacity is based primarily on the clinician's interpretation of the person's reason for his or her decision, then the clinician should seek further input from others, such as the patient's family or relevant representatives from the patient's cultural or religious group. If the clinician suspects that a decision is based substantially on delusions or depression, then psychiatric evaluation is recommended.

Mr. G's clinician notes that the patient has no known allergies and has taken penicillin in the past. The clinician explains that the pills are to treat the sore throat but may cause diarrhea or a rash. The clinician asks Mr. G to review the information to ensure that everything is clear. Mr. G says: "You're giving me these pills to help my throat. If I get diarrhea or any skin problems I should stop and let you know." The clinician concludes that Mr. G is able to understand the relevant information and to appreciate the reasonably foreseeable consequences of accepting treatment. Furthermore, the decision to accept is not based on a delusion, but on a desire for symptom relief. The entire capacity assessment takes less than 1 minute.

Mr. H's specific capacity assessment shows that he has the ability to understand his condition ("I have had a stroke to the left cerebellum, which has left me clumsy on the left side. It was caused by a blood clot from the heart"), the proposed treatment ("You want to thin my blood with warfarin"), the option of refusing ("I don't want it"), as well as the ability to appreciate the reasonably foreseeable consequences of refusing the treatment ("I might have another stroke without the pills, but I don't want them") and of accepting it ("You say that the pills might reduce the chance of stroke, but it can also cause bleeding"). Explaining the reason for his refusal, Mr. H says: "I think that the women who draw the blood are vampires. You want to thin my blood so it is easier for them to drink." Mr. H is subsequently evaluated by a psychiatrist, who diagnoses acute mania. Mr. H's wife later reveals that manic depressive disorder had previously been diagnosed, but Mr. H had stopped his lithium therapy several months before his stroke.

Mrs. I's specific capacity assessment showed that she had the ability to understand her condition ("My toes are dead. They are very smelly"), the proposed treatment ("You want to cut off my toes"), and the option of refusing ("I do not want you to cut them off"), as well as some ability to appreciate the reasonably foreseeable consequences of refusing ("You say I will die, but I don't know about this. I wonder what you will do with my toes after you cut them off. I don't really trust the doctors. I think they just want to give the students some practice"). Mrs. I reveals that she is a con-centration-camp survivor with a deep mistrust of physicians. She also says that 7 years ago when she had gangrene of the left foot and refused ampu-tation the foot had healed. Because the clinician remains unsure of Mrs. I's capacity and suspects depression, a psychiatric consultation is requested. Mrs. I admits to having a persistent depressed mood and several vegetative signs of depression. However, she denies feelings of hopelessness, guilt, persecution or worthlessness. Ultimately, Mrs. I is felt to be capable but depressed. She accepts treatment for depression. Her foot condition stabi-lizes and at 1 year of follow-up she is able to walk but still requires daily treatments for her foot.

Mr. J is re-evaluated 4 hours later, at which time he has gained maximum benefit from the medication for his Parkinson's disease. At this time, he is able to communicate and answer questions, and is clearly capable.

References

1. Sharpe G. Consent and minors. *Health Law Can* 1993;13:197-207.
2. *Hospitals Management Regulations (EC653/93) pursuant to the Hospitals Act* RSPEI 1988, Cap H-10.
3. *Medical Consent of Minors Act*, RSNB 1973, c M-61, ss 2, 3(1), 3(2).
4. *Arts* 17-18 CCQ.
5. *Hospital Standards Regulations*, 1980, SR 331/79 as amended.
6. *Infants Act*, RSBC 1979, c 196, s 16(1).
7. Canadian Medical Association. Informed decision-making [policy summary]. *CMAJ* 1986;135:1208A.
8. Mebane AH, Rauch HB. When do physicians request competency evaluations? *Psychosomatics* 1990;31:40-6.
9. Katz M, Abbey S, Rydall A, Lowy F. Psychiatric consultation for competency to refuse medical treatment. *Psychosomatics* 1995;36:33-41.
10. Appelbaum PS, Roth LH. Patients who refuse treatment in medical hospitals. *JAMA* 1983;250:1296-301.
11. Molloy DW, Alemayehu E, Robert R. A standardized Mini Mental State Examination: its reliability compared to the traditional Mini Mental State Examination. *Am J Psychiatry* 1991;48:102-5.
12. Janofsky JS, McCarthy RJ, Folstein MF. The Hopkins Competency Assessment Test: a brief method for evaluating patients' capacity to give informed consent. *Hosp Community Psychiatry* 1992;43:132-6.
13. Fitten LJ, Waite MS. Impact of medical hospitalization on treatment: decision making capacity in the elderly. *Arch Intern Med* 1990;150:1717-21.
14. Fitten LJ, Lusky R, Hamann C. Assessing treatment decision-making capacity in elderly nursing home residents. *J Am Geriatr Soc* 1990;38:1097-104.
15. Rutman D, Silberfeld M. A preliminary report on the discrepancy between clinical and test evaluations of competence. *Can J Psychiatry* 1992;37:634-9.
16. Freedman M, Stuss DT, Gordon M. Assessment of competency: the role of neurobehavioral deficits. *Ann Intern Med* 1991;115:203-9.

17. Kaufmann CL, Roth LH, Lidz CW, Meisel A. Informed consent and patient decisionmaking: the reasoning of law and psychiatry. *Int J Law Psychiatry* 1982;4:345-61.

18. Markson LJ, Kern DC, Annas GJ, Glantz LH. Physician assessment of patient competence. *J Am Geriatr Soc* 1994;42:1074-80.

19. Etchells EE, Darzins P, Silberfeld M, Singer PA, McKenny J, Naglie G, et al. Assessment of patient capacity to consent to treatment. *J Gen Intern Med* 1999. In press.

20. Molloy DW, Silberfeld M, Darzins P, Guyatt GH, Singer PA, Rush B, et al. Measuring capacity to complete an advance directive. *J Am Geriatr Soc* 1996;44:660-4.

21. Gutheil TG, Appelbaum PS. *Clinical handbook of psychiatry and the law*. New York: McGraw-Hill; 1982.

22. Pruchno RA, Smyer MA, Rose MS, Hartman-Stein PE, Henderson-Laribee DL. Competence of long-term care residents to participate in decisions about their medical care: a brief objective assessment. *Gerontologist* 1995;35:622-9.

23. Ben-Aron MH, Hoffman BF. Patient competence to consent: a physician guide. *Ont Med Rev* 1989:56(4):8-12.

24. Hoffman BF, Srinivasan AJ. A study of competence to consent to treatment in a psychiatric hospital. *Can J Psychiatry* 1992;37:179-82.

25. Grossman L, Summers F. A study of the capacity of schizophrenic patients to give informed consent. *Hosp Community Psychiatry* 1980;31:205-6.

26. Bean G, Nishisato S, Rector NA, Glancy G. The psychometric properties of the competency interview schedule. *Can J Psychiatry* 1994;39:368-76.

27. Naglie G, Silberfeld M, O'Rourke K, Fried B, Corber W, Bombardier C, et al. A randomized trial of a decisional aid for mental capacity assessments. *J Clin Epidemiol* 1993;46:221-30.

28. Ganzini L, Lee MA, Heintz RT, Bloom JD, Fenn DS. The effect of depression treatment on elderly patients' preferences for life-sustaining medical therapy. *Am J Psychiatry* 1994;151:1631-6.

29. Sullivan MD, Youngner SJ. Depression, competence and the right to refuse lifesaving medical treatment. *Am J Psychiatry* 1994;151:971-8.

Acknowledgement: Ms. Sharon Smith for careful preparation of the manuscript.

Editor's note: The Aid to Capacity Evaluation is available on the University of Toronto Joint Centre for Bioethics Web site at www.utoronto.ca/jcb

4

Voluntariness

Edward Etchells, MD, MSc; Gilbert Sharpe, BA, LLB, LLM;
Mary Jane Dykeman, LLB; Eric M. Meslin, PhD; Peter A. Singer, MD, MPH

Mrs. K, who is 85 years old, was born in Germany but is fluent in English. She lives alone and carries out most activities of daily living independently. One day she collapses on her way to the grocery store. She is taken to hospital, where a large subarachnoid hemorrhage is diagnosed. She is comatose for 3 days. When she awakes on the third night she appears extremely confused and speaks only in German. She repeatedly climbs out of bed and pulls at her bladder catheter. The surgeon wonders if she should be physically restrained.

Mr. L is 65 years old and has been admitted to hospital with severe iron-deficiency anemia. After his condition is stabilized by means of a blood transfusion, an endoscopy is ordered. The attending physician tells Mr. L that he will "have a test" because "he must be bleeding from the bowel." He adds, "I want you to have this test before you go home." Mr. L, dressed in a hospital gown, is lying on a stretcher in the hallway outside the endoscopy suite when the endoscopist arrives.

Mr. M is 90 years old and lives with his wife in a seniors' apartment. He is independent in most activities of daily living. He is admitted to hospital with acute myocardial infarction complicated by mild congestive heart failure. The emergency physician discusses advanced cardiac life support (cardiopulmonary resuscitation [CPR], and electrical cardioversion and defibrillation). During the discussion, the clinician emphasizes that CPR causes broken ribs and, even when successful, leaves the patient with severe neurologic impairment. Mr. M declines CPR and is consequently admitted to a ward bed without continuous cardiac monitoring.

What is voluntariness?

In the context of consent, "voluntariness" refers to a patient's right to make treatment decisions free of any undue influence. A patient's freedom to decide can be impinged upon by internal factors arising from the patient or the patient's condition or by external factors. External factors, which are the focus of this chapter, include the ability of others to exert control over a patient by force, coercion or manipulation.[1] Force involves the use of physical restraint or sedation to enable a treatment to be given. Coercion involves the use of explicit or implicit threats to ensure that a treatment is accepted (e.g., "If you don't let us do these tests, then we will discharge you from the hospital!"). Manipulation involves the deliberate distortion or omission of information in an attempt to induce the patient to accept a treatment.[2,3] Mr. M is a manipulated patient: no reasonable person would consent to CPR if he or she believed that it always resulted in pain and severe brain damage, with no hope of any benefit.

The requirement for voluntariness does not imply that clinicians should refrain from persuading patients to accept advice. Persuasion involves appealing to the patient's reason in an attempt to convince him or her of the merits of a recommendation.[4] In attempting to persuade the patient to follow a particular course of action, the clinician still leaves the patient free to accept or reject this advice.

Why is voluntariness important?

Ethics

Voluntariness is an ethical requirement of valid consent. It is grounded in several related concepts, including freedom, autonomy and independence.[5] The goal of the consent process is to maximize the opportunity for decisions to be reached autonomously.[6] Practically, it requires the physician to ensure that situations do not arise in which the patient's actions are substantially controlled by others. There is an inherent power imbalance in the physician–patient relationship; clinicians should strive to minimize this imbalance by fostering autonomous decision-making by their patients. (The concept of "consent" is discussed in chapter 1.)

Law

Voluntariness is a legal requirement of valid consent. In *Beausoleil* v. *Sisters of Charity*[7] a young woman about to undergo spinal surgery repeatedly requested a general anesthetic and refused a spinal anesthetic. After the patient had been sedated, the anesthetist convinced her to have a spinal anesthetic. The patient was subsequently paralysed as a result of the procedure and successfully sued the anesthetist. In testimony, a witness said that the patient "refused [the spinal anesthetic], but they continued to offer it to her; finally she became tired and said: 'You do as you wish' or something like that."[8] The judge stated that the patient's agreement to the spinal anesthetic was involuntary, because it rested on "words which denote defeat, exhaustion, and abandonment of the will power."[8]

In *Ferguson* v. *Hamilton Civic Hospitals*[9] a patient unsuccessfully sued for battery after undergoing angiography that resulted in quadriplegia. Although the suit was unsuccessful, the court was critical of the circumstances in which the consent was obtained and suggested that "the informing of a patient should occur at an earlier time than when he is on the table immediately before undergoing the procedure."[10] It has been suggested that obtaining consent just before a major procedure is problematic, because "the setting and the immediacy of the medical procedure militate against a patient being able to make a free or voluntary decision."[11]

Some legislation allows for treatment to be given in certain circumstances without the patient's volition. For example, irresponsible people with communicable diseases may be treated against their objection, as in the case of patients with tuberculosis who are noncompliant with treatment. Also, all provinces allow for the involuntary admission of patients to psychiatric facilities, provided they present an immediate risk to themselves or others, or are unable to take care of themselves. However, in most provinces, a patient who is admitted involuntarily may not be treated without consent except in emergency situations in which the patient is incapable. (Patient "capacity" is discussed in chapter 3.) Because of the coercive nature of such circumstances, extra care should be taken in obtaining consent from patients who have been admitted involuntarily.

Policy

Voluntariness is an essential component of valid consent, and obtaining valid consent is a policy of the CMA[12] and other professional bodies.

Empirical studies

Psychiatric inpatients may be subject to explicit or implicit coercion even when their admission has been voluntary.[13-15] However, even patients who require involuntary admission can be given some measure of control over their situation by being allowed to choose the method of restraint.[16]

Institutionalization in nonpsychiatric hospitals or long-term care facilities can also be coercive. Even simple instructions to patients (e.g., "Don't get out of bed until after your breakfast") can give the patient a sense of diminished control.[17] Interventions that enhance the ability of long-term residents to exert control result in a greater sense of well-being,[18] and many long-term care facilities have developed successful programs to reduce the use of restraints.[19]

Outpatients are less likely than inpatients to be subjected to force and coercion,[20] but they may be susceptible to manipulation. Although we are unaware of any data on the frequency with which manipulation occurs, many studies indicate that decisions can easily by influenced by the manner in which information is presented.[21–24] It is possible for such manipulation to occur in clinical practice.

How should I approach voluntariness in practice?

Internal and external controlling factors can affect patients' decisions about treatment (Fig. 1). For example, a patient with metastatic prostate cancer and bone pain is subject to internal controlling factors. A symptom-free life without treatment is not possible, and the patient must make some decisions while suffering severe pain, at least until the pain is treated. These internal factors arise from the patient's medical condition rather than from an external source, such as any action by the clinician. The clinician's role is to minimize the potential controlling effect of these internal factors. For example, the clinician can reduce the impact of acute pain on decision-making by deferring nonurgent decisions until the pain has been treated.

External controlling factors may be related to the clinician, the health care setting or to other people such as family and friends. We will focus here

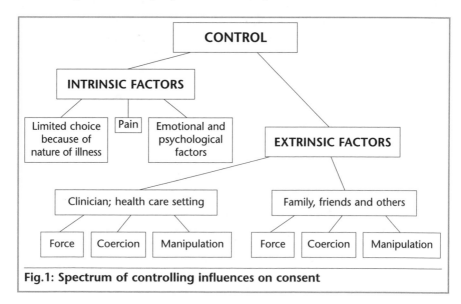

Fig.1: Spectrum of controlling influences on consent

on the clinician and the health care setting; the problems that can arise when family, friends or others exert excessive control are not discussed.

In the few circumstances in which it is acceptable for clinicians to use force, the least restrictive technique possible should be preferred. For example, if a patient is at immediate risk of harming himself or herself, simple observation in a supervised environment, rather than physical restraint or sedation, may be sufficient. Similarly, an elderly patient with delirium who is falling out of bed can be moved to a mattress on the floor so that the risk of falling is eliminated without physical restraint.

In psychiatric and long-term care institutions a patient advocate can help the clinician ensure that consent is not coerced.[25] Clinicians can also take steps to minimize the coercive nature of institutions by enhancing the patient's sense of choice. Useful strategies might include encouraging patients to involve their family in decisions, encouraging them to ask questions and promoting their awareness of the choices available to them (e.g., "I would like you to have a test tomorrow. Do you want to talk about it with your family? Is there any reason to delay?").

Clinicians can also take steps to minimize the potential for manipulation. First, because patients can be manipulated when the information they receive is incomplete, clinicians should ensure that adequate information has been disclosed to the patient. (The requirements for adequate disclosure are discussed in chapter 2.) Second, manipulation can occur when information is presented in a biased fashion. A useful strategy is to ask patients to review information in their own words. Also, if a patient who accepts therapy because of its potential benefits continues to accept it when its potential risks are emphasized, then the clinician can be more confident that this decision has not been manipulated.[26]

The surgeon tries to determine why Mrs. K is climbing out of bed. A German-speaking relative is contacted; she ascertains that Mrs. K is disoriented but is also very worried about her cat at home, who needs to be fed. The relative reassures Mrs. K that a neighbour has been feeding the cat. Mrs. K is visibly relieved and becomes less agitated. The surgeon decides that Mrs. K can be monitored safely without the bladder catheter, and the catheter is removed. The relative agrees to stay overnight to ensure that Mrs. K does not fall out of bed. Mrs. K is not restrained.

The endoscopist asks Mr. L to review the reasons for the test in his own words. Mr. L says that he's got "no choice but to have the test" because "my doctor needs it done before I go home." Because the endoscopy is not an emergency, the endoscopist calls the attending physician, who agrees that the test should be delayed. After a further discussion that afternoon, Mr. L consents to the endoscopy, which is performed the next morning.

On the medical ward, Mr. M's attending physician asks why he has refused advanced cardiac life support. Mr. M explains that if his heart stopped then he would "rather be dead than a vegetable with broken ribs." He adds that he hopes to be alive and able to attend his granddaughter's wedding next month. The clinician discusses the potential benefit of defibrillation in the event of a witnessed cardiac arrest related to acute myocardial infarction. Despite the potential benefits of CPR, Mr. M says he would prefer to forgo the treatment, because "I've lived a good life and I'm ready to go." He remains on the medical ward, recovers and attends his granddaughter's wedding.

References

1. Faden RR, Beauchamp TL. *A history and theory of informed consent.* New York: Oxford University Press; 1986. p. 259.
2. Pendleton DA, Bochner S. The communication of medical information in general practice consultations as a function of patients' social class. *Soc Sci Med* 1980;14A:669-73.
3. Shapiro MC, Najman JM, Chang A, Keeping JD, Morrison J, Western JS. Information control and the exercise of power in the obstetrical encounter. *Soc Sci Med* 1983;17:139-46.
4. Faden RR, Beauchamp TL. *A history and theory of informed consent.* New York: Oxford University Press; 1986. p. 261-2.
5. Faden RR, Beauchamp TL. *A history and theory of informed consent.* New York: Oxford University Press; 1986. p. 256-7.
6. Faden RR, Beauchamp TL. *A history and theory of informed consent.* New York: Oxford University Press; 1986. p. 239.
7. *Beausoleil* v. *Sisters of Charity* (1966), 56 DLR 65 (Que CA).
8. *Beausoleil* v. *Sisters of Charity* (1966), 56 DLR 65 at 76 (Que CA) note 7.
9. *Ferguson* v. *Hamilton Civic Hospitals* (1983), 23 CCLT 254 (Ont High Ct).
10. *Ferguson* v. *Hamilton Civic Hospitals* (1983), 23 CCLT 254 at 285 (Ont High Ct) note 10.
11. Picard E. *Legal liability of doctors and hospitals in Canada.* 2d ed. Toronto: Carswell, 1984:55.
12. Canadian Medical Association. Informed decision-making [policy summary]. *CMAJ* 1986;135:1208A.
13. Reed SC, Lewis DA. The negotiation of involuntary admission in Chicago's state mental hospitals. *J Psychiatr Law* 1990;18(spring/summer):137-63.
14. Kinzie JD, Holmes JL, Arent J. Patients' release of medical records. Involuntary, uninformed consent? *Hosp Community Psychiatry* 1985;36:843-7.
15. Rogers A: Coercion and "voluntary" admission: an examination of psychiatric patient views. *Behav Sci Law* 1993;11:259-67.
16. Sheline Y, Nelson T. Patient choice: deciding between psychotropic medication and physical restraints in an emergency. *Bull Am Acad Psychiatry Law* 1993;21:321-9.
17. Hewison A: Nurses' power in interactions with patients. *J Adv Nurs* 1995; 21:75-82.
18. Langer EJ, Rodin J. The effects of choice and enhanced personal responsibility for the aged: a field experiment in an institutional setting. *J Pers Soc Psychol* 1976;34:191-8.

19. Miles SH, Meyers R. Untying the elderly: 1989 to 1993 update. *Clin Geriatr Med* 1994;10:513-25.
20. Connelly JE, Campbell C. Patients who refuse treatment in medical offices. *Arch Intern Med* 1987;47:1829-33.
21. Mazur DJ, Hickam DH. The effect of physicians' explanations on patients' treatment preferences. *Med Decis Making* 1994;14:255-8.
22. Brun W, Teigen KH. Verbal probabilities: Ambiguous, context-dependent, or both? *Organ Behav Hum Decis Process* 1988;41:390-404.
23. Pepper S, Prytulak LS. Sometimes frequently means seldom: context effects in the interpretation of quantitative expressions. *J Res Pers* 1974;8:95-101.
24. Sutherland HJ, Lockwood GA, Tritchler DL, Sem F, Brooks L, Till JE. Communicating probabilistic information to cancer patients: Is there "noise" on the line? *Soc Sci Med* 1991;32:725-31.
25. Review of Advocacy for Vulnerable Persons. *You've got a friend: a review of advocacy in Ontario* [report]. Toronto: Ontario Ministry of the Attorney General; 1987. p. 52-8.
26. Redelmeier PA, Rozin P, Kahneman D. Understanding patients' decisions: cognitive and emotional perspectives. *JAMA* 1993;270:72-6.

Substitute decision-making

Neil M. Lazar, MD; Glenn G. Griener, PhD;
Gerald Robertson, LLB, LLM; Peter A. Singer, MD, MPH

Mr. N is a 35-year-old man with advanced AIDS in whom AIDS-related dementia has recently been diagnosed. When he was still capable he told his partner and close family members that if he ever "lost his mind" because of his HIV infection he would want to receive only comfort measures for any new medical problem. During the past 2 weeks Mr. N's caregivers have noticed that he is having increasing difficulty breathing. In view of his medical history they think he probably has a recurrence of *Pneumocystis carinii* pneumonia (PCP). A chest x-ray film shows probable PCP. The physician knows that Mr. N has had a lot of difficulty with adverse drug reactions in the past and wonders whether or not the patient should be admitted to hospital for further investigations and treatment.

Mr. O is an 85-year-old widower with Alzheimer's disease, which was diagnosed 10 years ago. His clinical condition has deteriorated, and he is no longer able to maintain an adequate energy intake by mouth. Feeding by nasogastric tube has been tried, but the patient repeatedly pulls out the tube. The option of using a surgically placed feeding tube is being considered by his caregivers. His family includes 5 adult children, all of whom are available. Two of them think their father would want the feeding tube, 2 others think he would not want it, and 1 does not know what he would want.

Mrs. P, a 73-year-old widow with advanced chronic obstructive pulmonary disease and osteoporosis, has recently moved into a nursing home because of deteriorating health. Her closest family members include 3 married children. One daughter lives in the same city, and the other 2 children live more than an hour away by car. Mrs. P's breathing deteriorates suddenly and she is transferred to hospital for assessment and treatment. When she is seen in the emergency department she is confused because of either respiratory failure or the toxic effects of an infection. Blood analysis reveals significant hypoxemia and respiratory acidosis. The attending physician wonders whether or not Mrs. P should be intubated. She has never required intubation before, and her hospital records give no instructions with regard to resuscitation. Mrs. P's daughter has just arrived and is waiting to talk to the physician.

What is substitute decision-making?

In theory, incapable patients have the same right to consent to diagnostic tests and treatments as do capable patients. In practice, however, incapable patients cannot exercise this right. Substitute decision-making is a means of making decisions about health care on behalf of patients who are incapable.

Why is substitute decision-making important?

Ethics

The primary ethical rationale for substitute decision-making is the principle of respect for autonomy.[1] It is an attempt, albeit an imperfect one, to extend the patient's control over his or her own health care. This rationale has a number of important practical implications.

First, the substitute decision-maker should be the person or persons with the best knowledge of the patient's specific wishes, or of the patient's values and beliefs, as they pertain to the present situation. In general, close relatives are preferred as substitute decision-makers in the belief that they will know the patient well enough to replicate the decision that the patient would make if he or she were capable. Of course, the patient may be estranged from his or her spouse, parents, children or siblings, and in some instances a friend or perhaps the patient's primary care physician or nurse will know the patient's wishes best.

Second, the task of substitute decision-makers is to decide not how they would want to be treated were they in the patient's situation but, rather, how the patient would want to be treated. Despite the best intentions and most sincere efforts of those involved, it sometimes remains a mystery what the patient would have chosen. When good information about the patient's wishes, or values and beliefs, is lacking, or when the available information is contradictory, the decision-maker may be forced to make a judgement as to the patient's best interest in the given circumstances.

Finally, when relatives disagree they should be encouraged to focus their attention on the question of what the patient would want to be done or what is in the patient's best interest.

Law

Nonstatutory law relating to substitute decision-making is rather uncertain. It is probably the case that family members do not have the legal power to make health care decisions on behalf of an incompetent adult patient and that only a court-appointed guardian, or the court itself, has that power.[2-4] In practice, of course, family members are often consulted and viewed as having decision-making authority. The Yukon Territory, British Columbia, Ontario, Quebec and Nova Scotia have recognized that this situation is unsatisfactory and have enacted legislation giving family members the right to make health care decisions on behalf of incompetent patients. British Columbia, Alberta, Manitoba, Ontario, Quebec, Nova Scotia and Newfoundland have passed legislation that enables individuals to designate the person they wish to make health care decisions for them once they are no longer able to make such decisions themselves. Because the applicable statutory and common law varies across Canada, it is advisable that practitioners become familiar with the legal requirements in their own province or territory.

Policy

Substitute decision-making is an important part of the health care policies of health care facilities and professional organizations.[5,6] For instance, the CMA policy on resuscitative interventions includes provisions related to substitute decision-making.[7]

Empirical studies

Studies have demonstrated that partners and close family members cannot accurately predict patients' preferences for life-sustaining treatments.[8-10] This should raise concern about uninformed substitute decision-making and encourage advance care planning. (Approaches to advance care planning will be discussed in chapter 6.)

How should I approach substitute decision-making in practice?

The process of substitute decision-making poses 2 important questions. First, who should make the decision for the incapable person? Second, how should the decision be made? Although the answer to these questions varies from one jurisdiction to another, the overall goal of substitute decision-making is to replicate the decision the patient would make if he or she were still capable.

The most appropriate person to act as substitute decision-maker is someone appointed by the patient while he or she is still capable, or by a proxy advance directive or by a court. Other substitute decision-makers, in their usual order of ranking, include the patient's spouse or partner, child, parent, sibling or other relative. In some jurisdictions a public official will serve as substitute decision-maker for a patient who has no such person available.

The criteria on which the decision should be based are the specific wishes previously expressed by the patient, the patient's known values and beliefs and the patient's best interests. The patient's wishes are those preferences expressed by the patient while he or she was competent that seem to apply to the decision that needs to be made. Some patients record their wishes in an advance directive. Values and beliefs are less specific than wishes but allow the substitute decision-maker to infer, in light of other choices the patient has made and his or her approach to life in general, what he or she would decide in the present situation. The calculation of a patient's best interests is based on objective estimates of the benefits and burdens of treatment to the patient.

The role of the health care professional is to facilitate the process of substitute decision-making by providing information that will enable the substitute to make an informed choice on the patient's behalf. Health care professionals should guide the substitute to consider the patient's previously expressed wishes, values and beliefs, or best interest (in this order). When it is apparent that the substitute is making a choice that is significantly different from what the patient might have chosen, health care providers find themselves in a difficult situation and should seek advice from colleagues, ethics committees and legal counsel.

Mr. N is incapable because of his AIDS-related dementia. The situation is not an emergency. The physician speaks to Mr. N's partner and close family members, who all agree that he would not want to be admitted to hospital to undergo any invasive procedures. They feel he would want to go home, perhaps with supplemental oxygen therapy to relieve some of his distress. They tell the physician that after his last episode of PCP Mr. N instructed them that he would never wish to go through the necessary treatment again. Palliative home oxygen therapy is arranged, and the patient dies 72 hours later.

Mr. O is permanently incapable because of his Alzheimer's disease. The problem is that his 5 children cannot agree on what treatment he would choose. In such situations, sensitive counselling with the family is needed; if this still does not resolve the conflict, referral to a board (e.g., the Consent and Capacity Board in Ontario) or to the courts might be required. As soon as the conflict with respect to who will make the decision for the patient is resolved, the proposed treatment can be discussed with that person. In this case, a social worker is able to bring the family together to reach a consensus as to which children are in the best position to act as substitute decision-makers. The patient dies from progressive Alzheimer's disease 6 months later without a feeding tube being placed.

Mrs. P is judged to be temporarily incapable. After discussing the patient's incapacity, the physician asks the daughter whether she knows what her mother would want if the situation deteriorates further. The daughter says that Mrs. P's quality of life declined after her husband died. Although she has never discussed this sort of situation directly with her mother, she does not think that her mother would want resuscitation. However, she is uncomfortable making this decision on her own. The physician suggests that she consult with her siblings. The physician says that in the meantime everything possible will be done to avoid intubation; however, intubation will proceed if it becomes medically necessary. Two hours later the daughter reports to the physician that all of the children feel that Mrs. P would refuse intubation if she were capable. Although the physician makes it clear that Mrs. P might be able to make this decision herself if she recovers from the current episode, the daughter requests that a "do not intubate" order be placed on the patient's chart. The physician agrees to write the order and plans to discuss it with the patient if her capacity improves.

References

1. Buchanan AE, Brock DW. *Deciding for others: the ethics of surrogate decision-making.* Cambridge (UK): Cambridge University Press; 1989.
2. Alberta Law Reform Institute. *Advance directives and substitute decision-making in health care.* Edmonton: The Institute; 1991. Report for discussion no 11.
3. Robertson GB. *Mental disability and the law in Canada.* 2nd ed. Toronto: Carswell; 1994.
4. Picard EI, Robertson GB. *Legal liability of doctors and hospitals in Canada.* 3rd ed. Toronto: Carswell; 1996.
5. Rasooly I, Lavery JV, Urowitz S, Choudhry S, Seeman N, Meslin EM, et al. Hospital policies on life-sustaining treatments and advance directives in Canada. *CMAJ* 1994;150:1265-70.
6. Choudhry NK, Ma J, Rasooly I, Singer PA. Long-term care facility policies on life-sustaining treatments and advance directives. *J Am Geriatr Soc* 1994;42:1150-3.
7. Joint statement on resuscitative interventions (update 1995). *CMAJ* 1995;153:1652A-1652C.
8. Emanuel EJ, Emanuel LL. Proxy decision-making for incompetent patients: an ethical and empirical analysis. *JAMA* 1992;267:2067-71.
9. Tsevat J, Cook EF, Green ML, Matchar DB, Dawson NV, Broste SK, et al. Health values of the seriously ill. *Ann Intern Med* 1995;122:514-20.
10. Seckler AB, Meier DE, Mulvihill M, Paris BE. Substituted judgment: How accurate are proxy predictions? *Ann Intern Med* 1991;115:92-8.

6

Advance care planning

Peter A. Singer, MD, MPH; Gerald Robertson, LLB, LLM;
David J. Roy, STL, PhL, DrTheol

> Mrs. Q is 63 years old and has no significant history of illness. She presents for a routine visit to her family physician. She recently read a newspaper article about a new law on living wills and wants to obtain some advice about them.
>
> Mr. R is a 40-year-old man with HIV infection diagnosed 2 years ago. He presents to an internist with symptoms of early dementia. The internist considers what Mr. R should be told about advance directives.

What is advance care planning?

Advance care planning is a process whereby a patient, in consultation with health care providers, family members and important others, makes decisions about his or her future health care.[1] This planning may involve the preparation of a written advance directive.[2,3] Completed by the patient when he or she is capable, the advance directive is invoked in the event that the patient becomes incapable. (The question of capacity is discussed in chapter 3.) Advance directives indicate whom the patient would want to make treatment decisions on his or her behalf and what interventions the patient would or would not want in various situations.

Why is advance care planning important?

Ethics

Advance care planning helps to ensure that the norm of consent is respected when sick people are no longer able to discuss their treatment options with physicians and thereby exercise control over the course of their care. This norm is grounded in the principle of self-determination and respect for autonomy, a classic expression of which is Justice Benjamin Cardozo's statement in 1914 that "Every human being of adult years and sound mind has the right to determine what shall be done with his own body."[4]

Although the principle of self-determination places high value on individual liberty, the usefulness of advance care planning is not limited to those whose world-view valorizes individualism. Advance care planning also rests on the principle of respect for persons, and this respect must extend to those whose cultural values emphasize the interdependence of human beings and the well-being of the family or community as a whole. Advance care planning recognizes that sick people suffer a loss of dignity when they cannot command respect for their considered and cherished intentions and that such intentions may be shaped by cultural values.

Advance care planning cannot avert all ethical uncertainties and conflicts in clinical decision-making. Some patients change their views as time passes, and others request life-prolonging interventions that subsequently prove to be unrealistic. Moreover, substitute decision-makers are not always sure that a patient's situation is equivalent to that described in an advance directive.

Law

British Columbia,[5] Alberta,[6] Saskatchewan,[7] Manitoba,[8] Ontario,[9,10] Quebec,[11] Nova Scotia,[12] Prince Edward Island[13] and Newfoundland[14] have legislation supporting the use of advance directives. (In British Columbia and Prince Edward Island this law has not yet been proclaimed.) An advance directive is referred to in law by various names: "representation agreement" (British Columbia), "personal directive" (Alberta), "health care directive" (Manitoba), "power of attorney for personal care" (Ontario), "mandate given in anticipation of ... incapacity" (Quebec), "consent agreement" (Nova Scotia) and "advance health care directive" (Newfoundland). The legislation varies from province to province with respect to the scope of advance directives, who can act as proxy for the patient, requirements for witnessing the advance directive, procedures for activating the advance directive, and so on. Physicians should familiarize themselves with the legislation in their province or territory. Even when there is no legislation, legal decisions such as that made in *Malette* v. *Shulman* and other cases[15-17] suggest that advance directives may still be legally valid.

Policy

The CMA supports the use of advance directives,[18] and some hospitals and long-term care facilities have policies regarding advance directives.[19,20]

Empirical studies

Key findings from empirical studies can be summarized as follows.

- Advance directives are generally viewed in a positive light by physicians and patients.[21–31] For example, 85% of family physicians in Ontario favoured the use of advance directives,[32] and 62% of medical outpatients wanted to discuss their preferences with regard to life-sustaining treatment.[33]
- 12% of Ontarians and 10% of Canadians have completed an advance directive form.[34,35]
- People change their preferences over time with respect to life-sustaining treatment.[36–38]
- Cultural values play an important role in advance care planning.[39,40]
- The implementation of programs to encourage advance care planning is associated with increased use of advance directives.[41–51]
- Few studies have been done on substitute decision-making for incapable persons with or without advance care plans and advance directives.[52–55]
- The effect of advance directives on health care costs has been the subject of debate.[56–60] Findings from the largest and most recent randomized trial do not support the hypothesis that the use of advance directives decreases health care utilization or costs.[61]

How should I approach advance care planning in practice?

Chapter 5 addressed the role of advance directives in substitute decision-making for incapable patients. In this chapter we focus on the process of planning care with capable patients.

The main goal of advance care planning is "to ensure that clinical care is shaped by the patient's preferences when the patient is unable to participate in decision making."[62] Moreover, it has recently been recognized that such planning is a social process that requires communication among all concerned; it is not simply the act of completing an advance directive form.[1,63]

The role of the physician in advance care planning is still being defined. Some authors believe that the physician's role is central. For example, Emanuel and associates[63] have described a framework for advance care planning within the context of the physician–patient relationship. This conception does not take into account the fact that many Canadians complete advance directives with the assistance of a lawyer in the context of estate counselling, or that over 2 million people requested Power of Attorney for Personal Care forms from the Office of the Public Guardian and Trustee after the Substitute Decisions Act was passed in Ontario.

Another view of advance care planning suggests that its primary goals are psychosocial ones (achieving a sense of control and relieving loved ones of the burden of decision-making) and that it occurs primarily outside the context of the physician–patient relationship.[64] Understanding advance care planning in a broader social context calls for a re-evaluation of the part that physicians and other health care providers have to play. If advance care planning occurs within families, for example, the physician should support that planning rather than direct it. The physician's primary role is that of educator. Physicians who raise the issue of advance care planning with patients who are unaware of their rights with respect to advance directives perform a valuable service. Patients who request assistance with advance care planning should first be directed to relevant information sources; these include documents provided by provincial governments, self-help publications such as *Let Me Decide*[65] and the *Living Will* of the University of Toronto Joint Centre for Bioethics.

Once a patient has obtained general information about advance care planning, the physician can help him or her to tailor an advance directive to the particular health situation of concern. Compared with the "generic" approach of preprinted advance directive forms, a "disease-specific" approach is less hypothetical and can be based on more precise prognostic information.[66] For instance, a physician caring for a patient with severe chronic obstructive pulmonary disease could draw the patient's attention to the issue of intubation and ventilation in the event of respiratory failure.

The physician can also ensure that the patient has correctly interpreted the information contained in a preprinted advance directive and is capable of completing it.[67,68]

Lawyers can make an important contribution by ensuring that an advance directive conforms to provincial legislation and is consistent with the patient's overall planning with regard to future incapacity and death. (This may involve other matters such as designating power of attorney for finances and preparing an estate will.)

Counselling is a valuable component of advance care planning. Whether such counselling is best performed by a physician, lawyer, nurse, social worker or other educator is unknown.

Physicians should suggest that patients review their advance care plans when their health status changes. This will help to ensure that the patient's preferences as expressed in an advance directive are current and likely to apply to future treatment decisions.

When the patient becomes incapable and his or her advance directive takes effect, the physician will seek consent to proceed with the proposed treatment plan from the substitute decision-maker appointed in the advance directive, as discussed in chapter 5.

Mrs. Q is requesting information about advance care planning. Her physician should refer her to one of the available information sources and encourage her to begin the process of advance care planning with her preferred substitute decision-maker. After a period of time, Mrs. Q and her substitute might together meet with the physician. At this meeting, the physician can review Mrs. Q's treatment preferences to ensure that she has understood the information in the advance directive form and is capable of completing it. If Mrs. Q is concerned about the legal validity of her advance directive, the physician might recommend that she consult a lawyer. If her health situation changes, the physician should recommend that Mrs. Q update her advance directive.

Mr. R, unfortunately, may soon be incapable of making health care decisions. The physician should raise the subject of advance care planning with him in a sensitive manner and follow the same steps as described for Mrs. Q. However, in the case of Mr. R, the physician will have to pay particular attention to the issue of capacity. This situation also represents an opportunity for the physician to tailor the information considered by Mr. R in advance care planning to the likely future: progressive cognitive deterioration.

References

1. Teno JM, Nelson HL, Lynn J. Advance care planning: priorities for ethical and empirical research. *Hastings Cent Rep* 1994;Nov-Dec:32S-36S.
2. Advance Directives Seminar Group, Centre for Bioethics, University of Toronto. Advance directives: Are they an advance? *CMAJ* 1992;146:127-34.
3. Emanuel L. Advance directives: What have we learned so far? *J Clin Ethics* 1993;4:8-15.
4. Cited in Faden RR, Beauchamp TL, King NMP. *A history and theory of informed consent.* New York: Oxford University Press; 1986. p. 123.
5. *Representation Agreement Act,* SBC 1993, c 67.
6. *Personal Directives Act,* SA 1996, c P-4.03.
7. *Health Care Directives and Substitute Health Care Decision Makers Act,* SS 1997, c. H-0.001.
8. *Health Care Directives and Consequential Amendments Act,* SM 1992, c 33.
9. *Health Care Consent Act,* SO 1996, c 31.
10. *Substitute Decisions Act,* SO 1992, c 30, as am by 1994, c 27, ss 43(2), 62; 1996, c 2, ss 3-60.
11. Art 12 CCQ.
12. *Medical Consent Act,* RSNS 1989, c 279.
13. *Consent to Treatment and Health Care Directives Act,* SPEI 1996, c 10.

14. *Advanced Health Care Directives Act*, SN 1995, c A-4.1.
15. *Malette* v. *Shulman* (1990), 67 DLR (4th) 321 (Ont CA).
16. *Airedale NHS Trust* v. *Bland*, [1993] AC 789 (HL).
17. Picard EI, Robertson GB. *Legal liability of doctors and hospitals in Canada.* 3rd ed. Toronto: Carswell; 1996. p. 67.
18. Canadian Medical Association. Advance directives for resuscitation and other life-saving or sustaining measures [policy summary]. *CMAJ* 1992;146:1072A.
19. Rasooly I, Lavery JV, Urowitz S, Choudhry S, Seeman N, Meslin EM, et al. Hospital policies on life-sustaining treatments and advance directives in Canada. *CMAJ* 1994;150:1265-70.
20. Choudhry NK, Ma J, Rasooly I, Singer PA. Long-term care facility policies on life-sustaining treatments and advance directives. *J Am Geriatr Soc* 1994;42:1150-3.
21. Kelner MJ, Bourgeault IL. Patient control over dying: responses of health care professionals. *Soc Sci Med* 1993;36:757-65.
22. Lo B, McLeod GA, Saika G. Patient attitudes to discussing life-sustaining treatment. *Arch Intern Med* 1986;146:1613-5.
23. Shmerling RH, Bedell SE, Lilienfeld A, Delbanco TL. Discussing cardiopulmonary resuscitation: a study of elderly outpatients. *J Gen Intern Med* 1988;3:317-21.
24. Frankl D, Oye RK, Bellamy PE. Attitudes of hospitalized patients toward life-support: a survey of 200 medical inpatients. *Am J Med* 1989;86:645-8.
25. Teno J, Fleishman J, Brock DW, Mor V. The use of formal prior directives among patients with HIV-related disease. *J Gen Intern Med* 1990;5:490-4.
26. Stolman CJ, Gregory JJ, Dunn D, Levine JL. Evaluation of patient, physician, nurse and family attitudes toward do not resuscitate orders. *Arch Intern Med* 1990;150: 653-8.
27. Gamble ER, McDonald PJ, Lichstein PR. Knowledge, attitudes and behaviour of elderly persons regarding living wills. *Arch Intern Med* 1991;151:277-80.
28. Emanuel LL, Barry MJ, Stoeckle JD, Ettelson LM, Emanuel EJ. Advance directives for medical care: a case for greater use. *N Engl J Med* 1991;324:889-95.
29. Joos SK, Reuler JB, Powell JL, Hickam DH. Outpatients' attitudes and understanding regarding living wills. *J Gen Intern Med* 1993;8:259-63.
30. Pfeifer MP, Sidorov JE, Smith AC, Boero JF, Evans AT, Settle MB, for the EOL [End of Life] Study Group. The discussion of end-of-life medical care by primary care patients and their physicians: a multicenter study using structured qualitative interviews. *J Gen Intern Med* 1994;9:82-8.
31. Molloy DW, Guyatt G, Elemayheu E, McIlroy WE. Treatment preferences, attitudes toward advance directives and concerns about health care. *Humane Med* 1991;7:285-90.
32. Hughes DL, Singer PA. Family physicians' attitudes toward advance directives. *CMAJ* 1992;146:1937-44.
33. Sam M, Singer PA. Canadian outpatients and advance directives: poor knowledge, little experience, but positive attitudes. *CMAJ* 1993;148:1497-502.
34. Singer PA, Choudhry S, Armstrong J. Public opinion regarding consent to treatment. *J Am Geriatr Soc* 1993;41:112-6.
35. Singer PA, Choudhry S, Armstrong J, Meslin EM, Lowy FH. Public opinion regarding end of life decisions: influence of prognosis, practice and process. *Soc Sci Med* 1995;41:1517-21.
36. Danis M, Garrett J, Harris R, Patrick DL. Stability of choices about life-sustaining treatment. *Ann Intern Med* 1994;120:567-73.
37. Emanuel LL, Emanuel EJ, Stoeckle JD, Hummel LR, Barry MJ. Advance directives: stability of patients' treatment choices. *Arch Intern Med* 1994;154:209-17.

38. Kohut N, Sam M, O'Rourke K, MacFadden DK, Salit I, Singer PA. Stability of treatment preferences; although most preferences do not change, most people change some of their preferences. *J Clin Ethics* 1997;8:124-35.
39. Caralis PV, Davis B, Wright K, Marcial E. The influence of ethnicity and race on attitudes toward advance directives, life-prolonging treatments, and euthanasia. *J Clin Ethics* 1994;4:155-65.
40. Blackhall LJ, Murphy ST, Frank G, Michel V, Azen S. Ethnicity and attitudes towards patient autonomy. *JAMA* 1995;274:820-5.
41. Sachs GA, Stocking CB, Miles SH. Empowerment of the older patient? A randomized controlled trial to increase discussion and use of advance directives. *J Am Geriatr Soc* 1992;40:269-73.
42. High DM. Advance directives and the elderly: a study of intervention strategies to increase use. *Gerontologist* 1993;33:342-9.
43. Rubin SM, Strull WM, Fialkow MF, Weiss SJ, Lo B. Increasing the completion of the durable power of attorney for health care: a randomized, controlled trial. *JAMA* 1994;271:209-12.
44. Hare J, Nelson C. Will outpatients complete living wills? A comparison of two interventions. *J Gen Intern Med* 1991;6:41-6.
45. Emanuel EJ, Weinberg DS, Gonin R, Hummel LR, Emanuel LL. How well is the Patient Self-Determination Act working? An early assessment. *Am J Med* 1993;95:619-28.
46. Silverman HJ, Tuma P, Schaeffer MH, Singh B. Implementation of the Patient Self-Determination Act in a hospital setting. *Arch Intern Med* 1995;155:502-10.
47. Markson LJ, Fanale J, Steel K, Kern D, Annas G. Implementing advance directives in the primary care setting. *Arch Intern Med* 1994;154:2321-7.
48. Luptak MK, Boult C. A method for increasing elders' use of advance directives. *Gerontologist* 1994;34:409-12.
49. Cohen-Mansfield J, Rabinovich BA, Lipson S, Fein A, Gerber B, Weisman S, et al. The decision to execute a durable power of attorney for health care and preferences regarding the utilization of life-sustaining treatments in nursing home residents. *Arch Intern Med* 1991;151:298-304.
50. Cohen-Mansfield J, Droge JA, Billig N. The utilization of the durable power of attorney for health care among hospitalized elderly patients. *J Am Geriatr Soc* 1991;39:1174-8.
51. Hanson LC, Tulsky JA, Danis M. Can clinical interventions change care at the end of life? *Ann Intern Med* 1997;126:381-8.
52. Danis M, Southerland LI, Garrett JM, Smith JL, Hielema F, Pickard CG, et al. A prospective study of advance directives for life-sustaining care. *N Engl J Med* 1991;324:882-8.
53. Morrison RS, Olson E, Mertz KR, Meier DE. The inaccessibility of advance directives on transfer from ambulatory to acute care settings. *JAMA* 1995;274:478-82.
54. Lynn J, Teno JM, Phillips RS, Wu AW, Desbiens N, Harrold J, et al. Perceptions by family members of the dying experience of older and seriously ill patients. SUPPORT Investigators. Study to Understand Prognoses and Preferences for Outcomes and Risks of Treatment. *Ann Intern Med* 1997; 126:97-106.
55. Hanson LC, Danis M, Garrett J. What is wrong with end-of-life care? Opinions of bereaved family members. *J Am Geriatr Soc* 1997;45:1339-44.
56. Schneiderman LJ, Kronick R, Kaplan RM, Anderson JP, Langer RD. Effects of offering advance directives on medical treatments and costs. *Ann Intern Med* 1992;117:599-606.

57. Molloy DW, Guyatt G. A comprehensive health care directive in a home for the aged. *CMAJ* 1991;145:307-11.
58. Molloy DW, Urbanyi M, Horsman JR, Guyatt GH, Bedard M. Two years' experience with a comprehensive health care directive in a home for the aged. *Ann R Coll Physicians Surg Can* 1992;25:433-6.
59. Chambers CV, Diamond JJ, Perkel RL, Lasch LA. Relationship of advance directives to hospital charges in a medicare population. *Arch Intern Med* 1994;154:541-7.
60. Teno JM, Lynn J, Phillips RS, Murphy D, Youngner SJ, Bellamy P. Do formal advance directives affect resuscitation decisions and the use of resources for seriously ill patients? *J Clin Ethics* 1994;5:23-30.
61. The SUPPORT Principal Investigators. A controlled trial to improve care for seriously ill hospitalized patients: the Study to Understand Prognoses and Preferences for Outcomes and Risks of Treatment (SUPPORT). *JAMA* 1995;274:1591-8.
62. Teno JM, Nelson HL, Lynn J. Advance care planning: priorities for ethical and empirical research. *Hastings Cent Rep* 1994;Nov-Dec:33S.
63. Emanuel LL, Danis M, Pearlman RA, Singer PA. Advance care planning as a process: structuring the discussions in practice. *J Am Geriatr Soc* 1995;43:440-6.
64. Singer PA, Martin DK, Lavery JV, Thiel EC, Kelner M, Mendelsohn DC. Reconceptualizing advance care planning from the patient's perspective. *Arch Intern Med* 1998;158:879-84.
65. Molloy W, Mepham V. *Let me decide: the health care directive that speaks for you when you can't.* Toronto: Penguin Books; 1992.
66. Singer PA. Disease-specific advance directives. *Lancet* 1994;344:594-6.
67. Silberfeld M, Nash C, Singer PA. Capacity to complete an advance directive. *J Am Geriatr Soc* 1993;41:1141-3.
68. Molloy DW, Silberfeld M, Darzins P, Guyatt GH, Singer PA, Rush B, et al. Measuring capacity to complete an advance directive. *J Am Geriatr Soc* 1996;44:660-4.

Editor's note: The University of Toronto Joint Centre for Bioethics *Living Will*, its French and Italian translations, and its versions specific to cancer and HIV infection are available on the Centre's Web site at www.utoronto.ca/jcb.

7

Truth telling

Philip C. Hébert, MD, PhD; Barry Hoffmaster, PhD;
Kathleen C. Glass, LLB, DCL; Peter A. Singer, MD, MPH

Mr. S is 26 years old and has recently joined a family physician's practice. He had an episode last year of unilateral arm weakness and visual blurring without headache that resolved within 12 hours. He was referred to a neurologist, who did several tests. Mr. S was subsequently told not to worry about the episode and thought no more about it. He has had no similar episodes since. In his medical records is a letter from the neurologist to the previous family physician stating that Mr. S almost certainly has multiple sclerosis. In the letter the neurologist explains that in order to prevent excessive worry he does not inform patients in the early stages of multiple sclerosis of their diagnosis.

What is truth telling?

In the practice of medicine, truth telling involves the provision of information not simply to enable patients to make informed choices about health care and other aspects of their lives but also to inform them about their situation. Patients may have an interest in medical information regardless of whether that information is required to make a decision about medical treatment. Truth telling requires accuracy and honesty: as Cabot wrote at the turn of the century, physicians should strive to create a "true impression" in the mind of the patient.[1] Thus, truth telling requires that information be presented in such a way that it can be understood and applied. By contrast, deception involves intentionally leading another to adopt a belief that one holds to be untrue.[2]

Why is truth telling important?

Ethics

The covenant of trust between physician and patient is central to the practice of medicine.[3] The candid disclosure and discussion of information not only helps patients to understand and deal with what is happening to them but also fosters and helps to maintain trust. Patients should be told the truth because of the respect due to them as persons. Patients have a right to be told important information that physicians have about them.

Not telling the truth can harm patients in many ways. Patients who remain uninformed about their condition may fail to obtain medical attention when they should. They may also make decisions affecting their lives that they would not make if they were aware of their condition. In addition, telling patients their diagnosis early in the course of a serious illness such as multiple sclerosis can be helpful simply because "some people find comfort in the knowledge that physicians can name their problem."[4]

Not telling patients the truth about their condition may entail deceiving them. Lack of candour or outright deception, even when well intentioned, can undermine the public's confidence in the medical profession.[5]

Law

Legal aspects of physician–patient communication are discussed in the chapters on consent (chapter 1) and on disclosure (chapter 2). Truth telling goes beyond disclosure for the purpose of assisting the patient in making treatment decisions and includes the broader notion of the accurate and honest communication of information. Canadian courts have dealt with lack of physician candour with regard to patient access to medical records, mishaps occurring in the course of treatment and the practice of "shielding" patients from bad news.

In discussing the right of patients to gain access to their own medical records, the Supreme Court of Canada acknowledged that information can have value to patients for its own sake and that "nondisclosure can itself affect the patient's well-being."[6] Good communication is required after treatment as well as before. For example, failure to tell a patient about the accidental puncture of his spleen during a lung biopsy was held to breach the physician's duty to inform the patient, particularly because the patient had asked what had occurred during the procedure. The judge concluded that litigation arose from a "less than satisfactory physician–patient relationship" precipitated by the lack of candid interchange following the mishap.[7]

A physician was found negligent in a case involving nondisclosure to the patient of his risk of having acquired HIV infection from a transfusion.[8] A family physician's desire "not to worry" a pregnant woman with information about serious but unlikely risks to the fetus after she contracted chicken pox proved an ineffective defence in a negligence action taken by the woman.[9]

Indeed, many legal actions result from communication difficulties between physicians and their patients.[10] Some patients who sue report having felt rushed or ignored during visits;[11] patients who are dealt with in this way are less likely to have their informational needs met than those who are given the time and opportunity to voice their concerns.[12] Effective and timely communication is essential to good care and can reduce the risk of malpractice claims.[13]

Physicians may be unsure whether to provide patients with statistics related to a prognosis. A court in California found no negligence in a physician's failure to disclose the precise statistical risk of death within 5 years to a patient with pancreatic cancer before the patient gave consent for experimental therapy. The court did not find, "as a matter of law," that any *particular* type of information must be disclosed, but it adhered to "the patient-based standard of disclosure" whereby "adequate information" must be given to enable the patient to make "an intelligent choice."[14]

The Supreme Court of Canada has granted that there may be narrow exceptions to truth telling, for example when the patient's emotional condition is such that the disclosure of bad news could cause harm.[15,16] The most relevant test for nondisclosure is "whether the disclosure would in itself cause physical and mental harm to *this* patient."[17] Physicians should start from the assumption that all patients are able to cope with the facts, and reserve nondisclosure for cases in which more harm will result from telling the truth than from not telling it.

Policy

An updated CMA Code of Ethics insufficiently emphasizes the wider duty of truth telling. It simply recommends that physicians provide patients with whatever information that will, from the patient's perspective, have a bearing on medical care decision-making and communicate that information in a way that is comprehensible to the patient.[18]

Empirical studies
Physicians

In a landmark study conducted in 1961, 90% of a sample of 219 US physicians reported that they would not disclose a diagnosis of cancer to a patient.[19] Of 264 physicians surveyed almost 20 years later, 97% stated that they would disclose a diagnosis of cancer.[20] This indicates a complete reversal of professional attitudes toward truth telling, at least in the context of a diagnosis of cancer.

Cultural and professional mores appear to influence physicians' attitudes toward truth telling. In one study, US physicians who reported that they commonly tell cancer patients the truth said that they did so in a way that was intended to preserve "hope" and "the will to live," both valued notions in US society.[21] The findings of another study suggested that gastro-enterologists from southern and eastern Europe were less likely to be candid with patients than their North American counterparts.[22] Another recent study showed a wide variation in psychiatrists' practices with respect to truth telling in patients with dementia.[23]

Patients

The literature suggests that most patients want to be informed about their situation. For example, in a 1957 study involving 560 cancer patients and their families 87% of respondents felt that patients should be told the truth about their illness.[24] In a study done before any treatment existed for multiple sclerosis, many patients with the disease felt they had a right to know what was wrong with them. Some were angry about being asked why they wished to know. One wrote: "Do I have to explain why? Just so that I know."[25] A survey conducted in 1982 indicated that 94% of patients wanted to know everything about their condition, 96% wanted to be informed of a diagnosis of cancer and 85% wanted to be given a realistic estimate of their time to live, even if this were less than 1 year.[26] Similar results may be found in another study.[27] More recent studies showed that over 90% of patients wanted to be told a diagnosis of Alzheimer's disease[28] and that over 80% of patients with amyotrophic lateral sclerosis wanted to be given as much information as possible.[29] A study of community-dwelling older persons revealed that 80% would prefer to know if they had Alzheimer's disease.[30]

Attitudes toward disclosure can vary from one cultural context to another. For example, in one study a greater percentage of Korean-born patients preferred to be given less information than did US-born patients.[31] Also, family members tend to protect affected relatives from knowing bad news, although they themselves would like to be informed.[32] However, one study of cancer patients revealed that they wanted doctors to respect their views about disclosure, rather than those of their family, should the views differ.[33]

Outcomes

Truth telling increases patient compliance,[34] reduces the morbidity such as pain[35] associated with medical interventions and improves health outcomes.[36]

Informed patients are more satisfied with their care and less apt to change physicians than patients who are not well informed.[37]

Some studies suggest that truth telling can have negative consequences. For example, the diagnosis of hypertension may result in decreased emotional well-being and more frequent absence from work.[38] Some patients may consider suicide on being given the diagnosis of Alzheimer's disease.[30]

How should I approach truth telling in practice?

Truth telling can be difficult in practice because of medical uncertainty and the concern that bad news might harm the patient. It can also be difficult when medical error occurs and when the patient's family is opposed to truth telling.

The pervasive uncertainty in medicine can and should be shared with patients.[39] Telling patients about the clinical uncertainties and the range of options available to them allows them to appreciate the complexities of medicine, to ask questions, to make informed, realistic decisions and to assume responsibility for those decisions.

Predicting what information a patient will find upsetting, or foreseeing *how* upsetting certain information will be, can be difficult. Patients may indicate, explicitly or implicitly,[40] their desire not to know the truth of their situation. When such desires are authentic they should be respected.

It is possible to deliver the truth in a way that softens its impact; many books provide practical suggestions on telling bad news.[41,42] The truth may be brutal, but "the telling of it should not be."[43] Disclosure of devastating news like the presence of Alzheimer's disease should be done with great care, and patients who react badly to the news should be followed up closely.

Physicians should disclose the occurrence of adverse events or errors to patients[44] but should not suggest that they resulted from negligence. The admission of error is not an admission of substandard practice. Negligence is a finding made in court, not by physicians or their colleagues.

Telling the truth can defuse resentment on the part of the patient and reduce the risk of legal action.[45] People sometimes sue physicians out of a "need for explanation — to know how the injury happened and why."[46] Truth telling at the time of the misadventure can ensure that an injured patient seeks appropriate corrective treatment promptly. Such frankness may thus foster, rather than undermine, the patient's trust in physicians.

In some cultural settings patients with terminal illnesses may waive their right to know about their situation or transfer that right to family members.[47] Physicians should explore such waivers sensitively with their patients to ascertain whether they are authentic requests. Patients should be explicitly offered the opportunity to be told important information.[48] When a patient has a serious illness such as cancer, it may be helpful to document his or her preferences regarding the involvement of family members. Families who resist disclosure of the truth should be counselled about the importance of truth telling, much as they might be counselled about the appropriate management of any medical problem.

It is important to bear in mind that substantial variability exists within cultures and that cultural values can change. For example, in Japan, where medicine has traditionally been very paternalistic,[49] the National Cancer Centre decided in 1995 that cancer patients must be given a form describing their disease and various side-effects of treatment.[50] National surveys in Japan have revealed "a small but clear trend" toward the disclosure of a diagnosis of cancer.[51]

If the neurologist seriously considered multiple sclerosis as a likely or working diagnosis he was not justified in withholding this information from Mr. S. A general worry about causing anxiety is not sufficient to exempt a physician from his responsibility to tell the patient the truth. Physicians need not and should not wait for near-certainty before they disclose information to patients. If Mr. S is not told about his condition and makes a decision that he would not otherwise have made, his physicians would bear some moral responsibility and even legal liability for any untoward outcome that resulted. Likewise, Mr. S's physicians could be held responsible if he failed to avail himself of new and potentially beneficial treatments[52] were his condition to worsen.

References

1. Cabot RC. The use of truth and falsehood in medicine: an experimental study. *Am Med* 1903;5:344-9.
2. Bok S. *Lying: moral choice in public and private life.* New York: Vintage Books; 1979. p. 14.
3. Cassel C. The patient–physician covenant: an affirmation of Asklepios. *Ann Intern Med* 1996;124:604-6.
4. Martin R. Some ethical issues in disclosure of progressive diseases of the nervous system. *South Med J* 1978;71:792-4.
5. Bok S. *Lying: moral choice in public and private life.* New York: Vintage Books; 1979. p. 28.
6. *McInerney* v. *MacDonald*, [1992] 2 SCR 138.
7. *Stamos* v. *Davies* (1985), 52 OR (2d) 11 at 25-6 (Ont High Ct).
8. *Pittman Estate* v. *Bain* (1994), 112 DLR (4th) 257 (Ont Ct [Gen Div]).
9. Cited in Mitchell SG. Diseases contracted during pregnancy: reviewing a physician's duty to disclose the risks faced by the fetus. *Ont Med Rev* 1994;61(7):53-7.
10. Evans K. Report of General Counsel. *Canadian Medical Protective Association annual report.* Ottawa, 1995:23.
11. Hickson GB, Clayton EW, Entman SS, Miller CS, Githens PB, Whetten-Goldstein K, et al. Obstetricians' prior malpractice experience and patients' satisfaction with care. *JAMA* 1994;272:1583-7.
12. Entman SS, Glass CA, Hickson GB, Githens PB, Whetten-Goldstein K, Sloan FA. The relationship between malpractice claims history and subsequent obstetric care. *JAMA* 1994;272:1588-91.

13. Nolin C. Malpractice claims, patient communication, and critical paths: a lawyer's perspective. *Qual Manage Health Care* 1995;3:65-70.
14. *Arato* v. *Avedon*, 23 Cal Rptr 2d 131 at 140 (Cal Sup Ct 1993).
15. *Hopp* v. *Lepp*, [1980] SCR 192.
16. *Reibl* v. *Hughes*, [1980] 2 SCR 895.
17. Picard E. *Legal liability of doctors and hospitals in Canada*. 2nd ed. Toronto: Carswell; 1984. p. 99.
18. Canadian Medical Association. Code of ethics. *CMAJ* 1996;155:1176A-B.
19. Oken D. What to tell cancer patients: a study of medical attitudes. *JAMA* 1961;175:1120-8.
20. Novack D, Plumer R, Smith R, Ochtill H, Morrow G, Bennett J. Changes in physicians' attitudes toward telling the cancer patient. *JAMA* 1979;241:897-900.
21. Good M, Good B, Schaffer C, Lind S. American oncology and the discourse on hope. *Cult Med Psychiatry* 1990;14:59-79.
22. Thomsen O, Wulff H, Martin A, Singer PA. What do gastroenterologists in Europe tell cancer patients? *Lancet* 1993;341:473-6.
23. Rice K, Warner N. Breaking the bad news: What do psychiatrists tell patients with dementia about their illness? *Int J Geriatr Psychiatry* 1994;9:467-71.
24. Samp R, Curreri A. Questionnaire survey on public cancer education obtained from cancer patients and their families. *Cancer* 1957;10:382-4.
25. Elian M, Dean G. To tell or not to tell the diagnosis of multiple sclerosis. *Lancet* 1985;2:27-8.
26. President's Commission for the Study of Ethical Problems in Medicine. *Making health care decisions*. vol 1. Washington: US Government Printing Office; 1982. p. 69-111.
27. Meredith C, Symonds P, Webster L, Lamont D, Pyper E, Gillis CR, et al. Information needs of cancer patients in west Scotland: cross sectional survey of patients' views. *BMJ* 1996;313:724-6.
28. Erde E, Nadal E, Scholl T. On truth telling and the diagnosis of Alzheimer's disease. *J Fam Pract* 1988;26:401-4.
29. Silverstein M, Stocking C, Antel J, Beckwith J, Siegler M. ALS and life-sustaining therapy: patients' desires for information, participation in decision-making, and life-sustaining therapy. *Mayo Clin Proc* 1991;66:906-13.
30. Holroyd S, Snustad D, Chalifoux Z. Attitudes of older adults on being told the diagnosis of Alzheimer's disease. *J Am Geriatr Soc* 1996;44:400-3.
31. Blackhall LJ, Murphy ST, Frank G, Michel V, Azen S. Ethnicity and attitudes toward patient autonomy. *JAMA* 1995;274:820-5.
32. Maguire CP, Kirby M, Coen R, Coakley D, Lawlor BA, O'Neill D. Family members attitudes toward telling the patient with Alzheimer's disease their diagnosis. *BMJ* 1996;313:529-30.
33. Benson J, Britten N. Respecting the autonomy of cancer patients when talking with their families: qualitative analysis of semistructured interviews with patients. *BMJ* 1996;313:729-31.
34. Eraker S, Kirscht J, Becker M. Understanding and improving patient compliance. *Ann Intern Med* 1984;100:258-68.
35. Egbert L, Battit G, Welch C, Bartlett M. Reduction of postoperative pain by encouragement and instruction of patients. *N Engl J Med* 1964;270:825-7.
36. Stewart MA. Effective physician–patient communication and health outcomes: a review. *CMAJ* 1995;152:1423-33.
37. Kaplan S, Greenfield S, Gandek B, Rogers W, Ware J. Characteristics of physicians with participatory decision-making styles. *Ann Intern Med* 1996;124:497-504.
38. Macdonald LA, Sackett DL, Haynes RB, Taylor DW. Labelling in hypertension: a review of the behavioural and psychological consequences [review]. *J Chronic Dis* 1984;37:933-42.
39. Logan R, Scott P. Uncertainty in clinical practice: implications for quality and costs of health care. *Lancet* 1996;347:595-8.
40. Pisetsky D. The breakthrough. *Ann Intern Med* 1996;124:345-7.

41. Tate P. *The doctor's communication handbook*. Oxford: Radcliffe Medical Press; 1995.
42. Buckman R. *How to break bad news*. Baltimore: Johns Hopkins University Press; 1992.
43. Jonsen A, Siegler M, Winslade W. *Clinical ethics*. 3rd ed. New York: McGraw-Hill; 1992. p. 53.
44. Picard EI, Robertson GB. *Legal liability of doctors and hospitals in Canada*. 3rd ed. Toronto: Carswell; 1996. p. 170-2.
45. Ritchie J, Davies S. Professional negligence: A duty of candid disclosure? *BMJ* 1995;310:888-9.
46. Vincent C, Young M, Phillips A. Why do people sue doctors? A study of patients and relatives taking legal action. *Lancet* 1994;343:1609-13.
47. Surbone A. Letter from Italy: truth telling to the patient. *JAMA* 1992;268:1661-2.
48. Freedman B. Offering truth: one ethical approach to the uninformed cancer patient. *Arch Intern Med* 1993;153:572-6.
49. Asai A, Fukuhara S, Lo B. Attitudes of Japanese and Japanese-American physicians towards life-sustaining treatment. *Lancet* 1995;346:356-9.
50. Ross C. Progress for patients amid Japan's uncertainty. *Lancet* 1995;345:1111-2.
51. Uchitomi Y, Yamawaki S. Truth-telling practice in cancer care in Japan. In: Surbone A, Zwitter M, editors. *Communication with the cancer patient: information and truth*. New York: New York Academy of Sciences; 1997. p. 290-9.
52. McDonald W. New treatments for multiple sclerosis. *BMJ* 1995;310:345-6.

Acknowledgements: Dr. Audrey Karlinsky for the case of Mr. S, and A. Mete, Program Assistant, Clinical Ethics Centre, Sunnybrook Health Science Centre, for help in preparing the manuscript.

8

Confidentiality

Irwin Kleinman, MD; Françoise Baylis, PhD;
Sanda Rodgers, LLB/BCL, LLM; Peter A. Singer, MD, MPH

Mr. T is 35 years old and is married. He has had unprotected sex with prostitutes on 2 occasions. Although he is asymptomatic, he becomes anxious about the possibility of having contracted a venereal disease and consults his physician. After conducting a thorough physical examination and providing appropriate counselling, Mr. T's physician orders a number of tests. The only positive result is for the HIV blood test. The physician offers to meet with Mr. T and his wife to assist with the disclosure of this information, but Mr. T states that he does not want his wife to know about his condition.

Mr. U is a 42-year-old professional who is living with his 14-year-old son and is involved in an acrimonious divorce. He is receiving drug therapy and weekly psychotherapy sessions for depression. Mr. U tells his psychiatrist that his wife makes him so crazy that at times he wants to kill her. He is concerned that in the heat of a confrontation he might act on this impulse. However, he recognizes that killing his wife would be devastating to his son, for whom he feels a great deal of affection and devotion.

Ms. V is 29 years old and has epilepsy. Her driver's licence was revoked when the ministry of transportation was notified of her history of seizures. Ms. V mentions in passing to her physician that she sometimes drives short distances to get groceries with her 3-year-old daughter in the car. When the physician challenges her about this, Ms. V emphasizes that her seizures are very infrequent. Finally, the physician states that he might be obliged to notify the authorities. Ms. V asks what more the authorities could do, now that they have revoked her licence. Would they put a police cruiser outside her house to make sure she doesn't drive?

What is confidentiality?

Physicians are obliged to keep information about their patients confidential. Confidentiality provides a foundation for trust in the therapeutic relationship.

Why is confidentiality important?

Ethics

Without an understanding that their disclosures will be kept secret, patients may withhold personal information. This can hinder physicians in their efforts to provide effective interventions or to pursue certain public health goals. For example, some patients may not feel secure in confiding a drug or alchohol dependence and thus may not have the benefit of treatment. Others may refrain from disclosing information that could alert the physician to the potential for harm or violence to others.

Respect for the confidentiality of patient information is not based solely on therapeutic considerations or social utility, however. Of equal, if not greater, importance is the physician's duty to respect patient autonomy in medical decision-making. Competent patients have the right to control the use of information pertaining to themselves. They have the right to determine the time and manner in which sensitive information is revealed to family members, friends and others.

In our strongly individualistic society the principle of autonomy is taken very seriously. This principle, however, is not absolute. As John Stuart Mill observed in the 19th century, personal freedom may legitimately be constrained when the exercise of such freedom places others at risk:

> The sole end for which mankind are warranted, individually or collectively, in interfering with the liberty of action of any of their number, is self-protection . . . [T]he only purpose for which power can be rightfully exercised over any member of a civilized community, against his will, is to prevent harm to others.[1]

Applied to the question of confidentiality, this suggests that although patients have the right to control how information about themselves is shared, this right is limited by the obligation not to harm others. When harm is threatened, the principle of autonomy (and hence the duty to preserve confidentiality) no longer takes precedence, and disclosure without the patient's authorization may be permissible or required.

Law

The confidentiality of patient information is prescribed in law. For example, physicians in Ontario are prohibited from providing information to third parties regarding a patient's condition or any professional service performed for a patient without the consent of the patient or his or her authorized agent unless such disclosure is required by law.[2] A breach of confidentiality that is not required by law may prompt disciplinary action by the College of Physicians and Surgeons of Ontario. Similar provisions concerning confidentiality exist in other provinces. Moreover, a breach of confidentiality may result in a civil suit.

Legal requirements to reveal certain kinds of information without the patient's consent are defined in both statutory and common law. The most notable legislated requirement involves the mandatory reporting of patients who suffer from designated diseases, those deemed not fit to drive and those suspected of child abuse.[3]

The case of *Tarasoff* v. *Regents of the University of California*[4,5] involved a psychologist who had reason to believe that his patient would kill a woman named Ms. Tarasoff. At the psychologist's request the campus police arrested the patient, but he was released when he assured the police that he would stay away from Tarasoff. No further action was taken, and the patient killed Tarasoff 2 months later.[4] Two decisions resulted from this case. The first established the duty to warn.[4] The American Psychiatric Association lobbied for the case to be reheard by the California Supreme Court.[6] As a result, a duty to protect was established that may or may not include a warning to the potential victim or the police.[5] The decision also implied that committing a dangerous patient to institutional care would obviate the need to warn.

Although the Tarasoff decision does not impose a legal duty upon Canadian physicians it could reasonably be expected that Canadian courts would apply similar reasoning in a comparable case. In *Tanner* v. *Norys* the Alberta Court of Appeal stated that if it were presented with a case involving a psychiatrist who failed to warn another of the risk of harm, then it would follow the reasoning used in the Tarasoff case.[7] In the report of the Commission of Inquiry into the Confidentiality of Health Information, Justice Horace Krever wrote that "it cannot be said with certainty that an Ontario court would decide a case involving identical circumstances [to those in *Tarasoff*] in a different way."[8]

Most recently, the College of Physicians and Surgeons of Ontario accepted recommendations formulated by an expert panel representing provincial and national medical organizations. The panel determined that physicians have a duty to warn when a patient reveals that he or she intends to do serious harm to someone else and it is more likely than not that this intention will be carried out.[9] The college has recommended that a standard of practice be established such that failure to warn would become a basis for a disciplinary finding of professional misconduct.[10]

Policy

The Hippocratic Oath[11] explicitly demands confidentiality in physicians' dealings with patients:

> What I may see or hear in the course of the treatment or even outside of the treatment in regard to the life of men, which on no account one must spread abroad, I will keep to myself holding such things shameful to be spoken about.[11]

The Hippocratic Oath and subsequent codes of ethics[12] admitted no exceptions to the duty of confidentiality. However, more recent codes allow that breaches of confidentiality may be justified or required in certain circumstances. For example, the CMA Code of Ethics states:

> Respect the patient's right to confidentiality except when this right conflicts with your responsibility to the law, or when the maintenance of confidentiality would result in a significant risk of substantial harm to others or to the patient if the patient is incompetent; in such cases, take all reasonable steps to inform the patient that confidentiality will be breached.[13]

Thus, according to the CMA Code of Ethics, physicians may disclose confidential information not only when they are required to do so by law but also when there is significant risk of substantial harm to others (which is, in effect, the reasoning underlying any legal duty to warn). The CMA position statement on AIDS advises physicians that

> disclosure to a spouse or current sexual partner may not be unethical and, indeed, may be indicated when physicians are confronted with an HIV-infected patient who is unwilling to inform the person at risk. Such disclosure may be justified when all of the following conditions are met: the partner is at risk of infection with HIV and has no other reasonable means of knowing the risk; the patient has refused to inform his or her sexual partner; the patient has refused an offer of assistance by the physician to do so on the patient's behalf; and the physician has informed the patient of his or her intention to disclose the information to the partner.[14]

The CMA has affirmed that medical records are confidential documents and that patient authorization is necessary for the disclosure of information contained in such records to a third party, unless such disclosure is required by law. Although medical records are the property of the physician or health care institution that compiled them, patients have the right to examine their records and to copy the information they contain.[15]

The Canadian Psychiatric Association[16] recommends that patients whom a physician believes at any point during treatment to be dangerous or potentially dangerous should be informed that confidentiality may be breached for his or her own protection and that of any potential victim. The association also recommends that any breach of confidentiality should be discussed beforehand and that the patient's cooperation should be enlisted if possible.

Empirical studies

Farber and associates[17] found that internal medicine residents based their decisions to breach confidentiality on factors other than the patient's intention to commit specific acts of violence. Reports of past violence, a criminal record and a history of high-cost crime increased the likelihood that confidential information would be disclosed. Cheng and collaborators[18] found that most adolescents who responded to their survey had problems that they wished to be kept secret and would not seek the help of health care professionals because of concerns about confidentiality. Ubel and colleagues[19] reported that inappropriate comments were made by hospital staff on 14% of elevator rides in the 5 institutions studied. Most frequently, these remarks constituted a breach of patient confidentiality.

How should I approach confidentiality in practice?

Physicians must respect their patient's confidences. Private information should be revealed to a third party only with the consent of the patient or his or her authorized representatives or when required by law.

Physicians should familiarize themselves with the legal requirements in their own province for the disclosure of patient information. When possible, it is important to discuss with the patient the necessity of any disclosure before it occurs and to enlist his or her cooperation. For example, it is helpful to persuade a patient suspected of child abuse to call the Children's Aid Society in the physician's presence to self-report, or to obtain his or her consent before the authorities are notified. This approach will prepare the way for subsequent interventions.

When harm is threatened and there is no specific legal requirement for disclosure the duty to warn may still override the duty to respect confidentiality. This is the case when the anticipated harm is believed to be imminent, serious (and irreversible), unavoidable except by unauthorized disclosure, and proportionate to the harm likely to result from disclosure. In determining the proportionality of these respective harms, the physician must assess and compare the seriousness of the harms and the likelihood of their occurrence. In all instances, but particularly when the harms appear equal, the physician must exercise his or her judgement. In cases of doubt, it would be prudent for the physician to seek expert advice, such as from the Canadian Medical Protective Association, before breaching confidentiality.

When a physician has determined that the duty to warn justifies an unauthorized disclosure, 2 further decisions must be made. Whom should the physician tell? How much should be told? Generally speaking, the disclosure should contain only that information necessary to prevent the anticipated harm and should be directed only to those who need the information in order to avert the harm. Reasonable steps should be taken to mitigate the harm and offense to the patient that may arise from the disclosure.

Mr. T's physician warns him that steps will have to be taken to ensure that his wife is made aware of his condition. These steps might include a direct warning to his wife and notification of the public health department. The physician subsequently decides to enlist the help of the department, which she believes to be experienced in dealing with this kind of issue. The public health authorities contact Mr. T and tell him that he must inform his wife. Mr. T responds to their authority and brings his wife to see his physician to be told about his condition.

Mr. U's psychiatrist carefully assesses the homicidal potential of his patient and concludes that Mr. U's wife is in no imminent danger. Mr. U does not really want to kill her and has never had violent outbursts in the past. More important, he does not want his son to suffer the negative consequences of such an action. Given the hostility he feels, Mr. U resolves to avoid contact with his wife. Psychotherapy continues, addressing a number of issues. A settlement with the wife is reached and Mr. U becomes involved in another relationship.

Ms. V's physician seeks legal advice to determine his obligations. He receives conflicting opinions. One opinion states that a duty to inform under these circumstances exists under the province's highway traffic act. A written opinion from the ministry of transportation states that once medical evidence has been received and action has been taken to suspend the driver's licence, further notification is not necessary. The relevant health care legislation permits confidentiality to be breached only when this is required by law.

This raises the question of whether the reasoning used in the Tarasoff case would apply, such that the physician has a duty to warn. The patient has had only 1 or 2 seizures during the past year and feels that she can tell when they are coming on. At most, she drives for 5 minutes 2 to 3 times per week. The probability of an accident resulting in serious irreversible harm is therefore very low. Furthermore, it is not clear that anyone is in a position to intervene even if notification were made.

Ms. V's physician feels that his patient is denying the reality of her illness and does not appreciate the risks involved. Over the next 2 weeks he continues to counsel her, explaining the risks to her daughter, to other people and to herself, given that she probably would not be insured in the event of an accident. This proves effective in penetrating Ms. V's denial of her illness. She tells the physician that she has decided not to drive again while her licence is revoked. Ms. V continues to work with her physician, addressing other areas of her life. This case highlights the importance of continuing to work therapeutically with patients while considering ethical and legal concerns.

References

1. Mill JS. On liberty. In: Robson JM, editor. *Essays on politics and society.* vol 1. Vol 18 of Robson JM, et al, editors, *Collected works.* Toronto: University of Toronto Press; 1977. p. 223.
2. O Reg 856/93, as am by 857/93; 115/94.
3. Evans KG. *A medico-legal handbook for Canadian physicians.* Ottawa: Canadian Medical Protective Association; 1990.
4. *Tarasoff* v. *Regents of the University of California,* 118 Cal Rptr 129, 529 P 2d 553 (Sup Ct 1974).
5. *Tarasoff* v. *Regents of the University of California,* 131 Cal Rptr 14, 551 P 2d 334 (Sup Ct 1976).
6. Mills MJ, Sullivan G, Eth S. Protecting third parties: a decade after Tarasoff. *Am J Psychiatry* 1987;144:68-74.
7. *Tanner* v. *Norys* (1980), 33 NR 355 (SCC); ref'g leave to appeal, [1980] 4 WWR 33 (Alta CA).
8. *Report of the Commission of Inquiry into the Confidentiality of Health Information.* vol 2. Toronto: Queen's Printer for Ontario; 1980. p. 432.
9. *Final recommendations of Ontario's Medical Expert Panel on the Duty to Inform.* Toronto: Institute for Clinical Evaluative Sciences in Ontario; 1996. p. A285-97.
10. *Duty to warn: report from council members' dialogue.* Toronto: College of Physicians and Surgeons of Ontario; 1996. p. 21-2.
11. Edelstein L. The Hippocratic Oath: text, translation and interpretation. In: Burns C, editor. *Legacies in ethics and medicine.* New York: Science History Publications; 1977. p. 12.
12. World Medical Association. International code of medical ethics (1949). In: *Encyclopedia of bioethics.* New York: Free Press; 1978. p. 1749-50.
13. Canadian Medical Association. Code of ethics. *CMAJ* 1996;155:1176A-B.
14. Canadian Medical Association. Acquired immunodeficiency syndrome [position statement]. *CMAJ* 1989;140:64A-B.
15. Canadian Medical Association. The medical record: confidentiality, access and disclosure [position statement]. *CMAJ* 1992;147:1860A.
16. Sharp F. Confidentiality and dangerousness in the doctor–patient relationship. The position of the Canadian Psychiatric Association. *Can J Psychiatry* 1985;30:293-6.
17. Farber NJ, Weiner JL, Boyer EG, Robinson EJ. Residents' decisions to breach confidentiality. *J Gen Intern Med* 1989;4:31-3.
18. Cheng TL, Savageau JA, Sattler AL, DeWitt TG. Confidentiality in health care: a survey of knowledge, perceptions, and attitudes among high school students. *JAMA* 1993;269:1404-7.

19. Ubel PA, Zell MM, Miller DJ, Fischer GS, Peters-Stefani D, Arnold RM. Elevator talk: observational study of inappropriate comments in public space. *Am J Med* 1995;99:190-4.

Editor's note: In *R. v. Cuerrier* [(1998), 127 CCC (3d) 1 SCC] the Supreme Court of Canada held that someone exposing sexual partners to HIV infection or other risk of serious injury without their knowledge does not have consent and is therefore convictable of sexual assault. This judgement is analogous to *Tarasoff* in that physicians may know of the direct risk a patient poses to others and therefore may have a legal duty of appropriate protection.

9

Involving children in medical decisions

Christine Harrison, PhD; Nuala P. Kenny, MD;
Mona Sidarous, LLB, LLM; Mary Rowell, MA, RN

> Eleven-year-old Wendy is a bright, loving child who was treated for osteosarcoma in her left arm. The arm had to be amputated, and Wendy was given a course of chemotherapy. She has been cancer-free for 18 months and is doing well in school. She is self-conscious about her prosthesis and sad because she had to give away her cat, Snowy, to decrease her risk of infection. Recent tests indicate that the cancer has recurred and metastasized to her lungs. Her family is devastated by this news, but her parents do not want to give up hope. However, even with aggressive treatment Wendy's chances for recovery are less than 20%.
>
> Wendy adamantly refuses further treatment. On earlier occasions she had acquiesced to treatment, only to struggle violently when it was administered. She distrusts her health care providers and is angry with them and her parents. She protests, "You already made me give up Snowy and my arm. What more do you want?" Her parents insist that treatment must continue. At the request of her physician, a psychologist and a psychiatrist conduct a capacity assessment. They agree that Wendy is probably incapable of making treatment decisions; her understanding of death is immature and her anxiety level very high. Nursing staff are reluctant to impose treatment; in the past Wendy's struggling and the need to restrain her upset them a great deal.

Why is it important to include children in medical decision-making?

Ethics

Traditionally, parents and physicians have made all medical decisions on behalf of children. However, just as the concept of informed consent has developed over the last 30 years with respect to competent adult patients, so new ways of thinking about the role of children in medical decision-making have evolved.

Ethical principles that provide guidance in the care of adults are insufficient in the context of caring for children.[1-3] Issues related to the voluntariness of consent, the disclosure of information, capacity assessment, treatment decisions and bereavement are more complex, as is the physician's relationship with the patient and the patient's family.[3,4] Adult models presume that the patient is autonomous and has a stable sense of self, established values and mature cognitive skills; these characteristics are undeveloped or underdeveloped in children.

Although it is important to understand and respect the developing autonomy of a child, and although the duty of beneficence provides a starting point for determining what is in the child's best interest, a family-centred ethic is the best model for understanding the interdependent relationships that bear upon the child's situation.[5] A family-centred approach considers the effects of a decision on all family members, their responsibilities toward one another and the burdens and benefits of a decision for each member, while acknowledging the special vulnerability of the child patient.

A family-centred approach presents special challenges for the health care team, particularly when there is disagreement between parent and child. Such a situation raises profound questions about the nature of the physician–patient relationship in pediatric practice. Integrity in this relationship is fundamental to the achievement of the goal of medicine,[6] which has been defined as "right and good healing action taken in the interest of a particular patient."[7] In the care of adults, the physician's primary relationship is with the particular capable patient. The patient's family may be involved in decision-making, but it is usually the patient who defines the bounds of such involvement.

The care of children, on the other hand, has been described in terms of a "triadic" relationship in which the child, his or her parents and the physician all have a necessary involvement (Dr. Abbyann Lynch, Director, Ethics in Health Care Associates, Toronto: personal communication, 1992). When there is disagreement between parent and child, the physician may experience some moral discomfort in having to deal separately with the child and parent.

The assumption that parents best understand what is in the interest of their child is usually sound. However, situations can arise in which the parents' distress prevents them from attending carefully to the child's concerns and wishes. Simply complying with the parents' wishes in such cases is inadequate. It is more helpful and respectful of the child to affirm the parents' responsibility for the care of their child while allowing the child to exercise choice in a measure appropriate to his or her level of development and experience of illness and treatment. This approach does not discount the parents' concerns and wishes but recognizes the child as the particular patient to whom the physician has a primary duty of care. This approach seeks to harmonize the values of everyone involved in making the decision.[6]

Law

The legal right to refuse medical treatment is related to, but not identical with, the right to consent to treatment. The patient's right to refuse even life-saving medical treatment is recognized in Canadian law[8,9] and is premised on the patient's right to exercise control over his or her own body. Providing treatment despite a patient's valid refusal can constitute battery and, in some circumstances, negligence.

To be legally valid the refusal of medical treatment must be given by a person deemed capable of making health care choices, that is, capable of understanding the nature and consequences of the recommended treatment, alternative treatments and nontreatment. In common law the notion of the "mature minor" recognizes that some children are capable of making their own health care choices despite their age.[10] In common law and under the statutory law of some provinces, patients are presumed capable regardless of age unless shown otherwise; in other provinces an age at which patients are presumed capable is specified (see chapter 3). When a child's capacity is in doubt an assessment is required.

In the case of children who are incapable of making their own health care decisions, parents or legal guardians generally have the legal authority to act as surrogate decision-makers. The surrogate decision-maker is obliged to make treatment decisions in the best interest of the child. Health care providers who believe that a surrogate's decisions are not in the child's best interest can appeal to provincial child welfare authorities. The courts have the authority to assume a *parens patriae* role in treatment decisions if the child is deemed to be in need of protection. This issue has arisen most commonly with respect to Jehovah's Witnesses who refuse blood transfusions for their children on religious grounds, and courts have authorized treatment in recognition of the state's interest in protecting the health and well-being of children.[11] Every province has child welfare legislation that sets out the general parameters of the "best interest" standard. Courts are reluctant to authorize the withholding or withdrawal of medical treatment, especially in the face of parental support for such treatment.

A special point to consider involves the use of patient restraints. The wrongful or excessive use of restraints could prompt an action of false imprisonment or battery. Restraint can involve the use of force, mechanical means or chemicals. The use of restraint compromises the dignity and liberty of the patient, including the child patient. Restraints should never be used solely to facilitate care but, rather, only when the patient is likely to cause serious bodily harm to himself or herself or to another. If restraint is required, the health care provider should use the least restrictive means possible, and the need for the restraint (as well as its effect on the patient) should be assessed on an ongoing basis.

Policy

The Canadian Paediatric Society has no policy regarding the role of the child patient in medical decision-making. The American Academy of Pediatrics statement on this question articulates the joint responsibility of physicians and parents to make decisions for very young patients in their best interest and states that "[p]arents and physicians should not exclude children and adolescents from decision-making without persuasive reasons."[12]

Empirical studies

As they grow, children develop decision-making skills, the ability to reason using complex concepts, an understanding of death[13] and the ability to imagine a future for themselves.[14] Children with a chronic or terminal illness may have experiences that endow them with insight and maturity beyond their years. Families often encourage children to participate in decision-making. Allowing even young children to make decisions about simple matters facilitates the development of skills that they will need to make more complex decisions later on.[15–17]

Because tools developed to assess the capacity of adults have not been tested with children, health care professionals working with children should be sensitive to the particular capacity of each child. Children are constantly developing their physical, intellectual, emotional and personal maturity. Although developmental milestones give us a general sense of capacities, 2 children of the same age will not necessarily have the same ability to make choices. Even when they are deemed capable of making health care choices, children need support for their decisions from family members and the health care team.

How should I determine the appropriate role of a child in medical decision-making?

Most children fall into 1 of 3 groups with respect to their appropriate involvement in decision-making.[18,19]

Infants and young children

Preschool children have no significant decision-making capacity and cannot provide their own consent. As surrogate decision-makers, parents should authorize (or refuse authorization) on their child's behalf, basing their decisions on what they believe to be in the child's best interest.

Primary-school children

Children of primary-school age may participate in medical decisions but do not have full decision-making capacity. They may indicate their assent or dissent without fully understanding its implications. Nonetheless they should be provided with information appropriate to their level of comprehension. Although the child's parents should authorize or refuse to authorize treatment, the child's assent should be sought and any strong and sustained dissent should be taken seriously.[20]

Adolescents

Many adolescents have the decision-making capacity of an adult.[21,22] This capacity will need to be determined for each patient in light of his or her
- ability to understand and communicate relevant information,
- ability to think and choose with some degree of independence,
- ability to assess the potential for benefit, risks or harms as well as to consider consequences and multiple options, and
- achievement of a fairly stable set of values.[23]

Many children and adolescents, particularly those who have been seriously ill, will need assistance in developing an understanding of the issues and in demonstrating their decision-making capacity. Age-appropriate discussions, perhaps with the assistance of teachers, chaplains, play therapists, nurses, psychologists or others skilled in communicating with children, are helpful. The child's participation may be facilitated by the use of art activities, stories, poems, role-playing and other techniques.[24,25]

Physicians should ensure that good decisions are made on behalf of their child patients. Although the interests of other family members are important and will influence decision-making, the child's interests are most important and are unlikely to be expressed or defended by the child himself or herself. Anxious, stressed or grieving family members may need assistance in focusing on what is best for the child. This may be especially difficult when a cure is no longer possible; in such cases a decision to stop treatment may seem like a decision to cause the child's death.

Whether or not the child participates, the following considerations should bear upon a treatment decision concerning that child:

- The potential benefits to the child
- The potential harmful consequences to the child, including physical suffering, psychological or spiritual distress and death
- The moral, spiritual and cultural values of the child's family

---

For Wendy, resuming aggressive treatment will have a serious negative effect on her quality of life. The chances of remission are small, yet a decision to discontinue treatment will likely result in her death. Because death is an irreversible harm, and decisions with serious consequences require a high level of competence in decision-making,[26] the capacity required would be very high. It has been determined that Wendy does not have this capacity.

Nevertheless, Wendy is included in discussions about her treatment options, and her reasons for refusing treatment are explored.[27] Members of the team work hard to re-establish trust. They and Wendy's parents come to agree that refusing treatment is not necessarily unreasonable; a decision by an adult patient in similar circumstances to discontinue treatment would certainly be honoured. Discussions address Wendy's and her parents' hopes and fears, their understanding of the possibility of cure, the meaning for them of the statistics provided by the physicians, Wendy's role in decision-making and her access to information. They are assisted by nurses, a child psychologist, a psychiatrist, a member of the clergy, a bioethicist, a social worker and a palliative care specialist.

Discussions focus on reaching a common understanding about the goals of treatment for Wendy. Her physician helps her to express her feelings and concerns about the likely effects of continued treatment. Consideration is given to the effects on her physical well-being, quality of life, self-esteem and dignity of imposing treatment against her wishes. Spiritual and psychological support for Wendy and her family is acknowledged to be an essential component of the treatment plan. Opportunities are provided for Wendy and her family to speak to others who have had similar experiences, and staff are given the opportunity to voice their concerns.

Ultimately, a decision is reached to discontinue chemotherapy and the goal of treatment shifts from "cure" to "care." Wendy's caregivers assure her and her family that they are not "giving up" but are directing their efforts toward Wendy's physical comfort and her spiritual and psychological needs. Wendy returns home, supported by a community palliative care program, and is allowed to have a new kitten. She dies peacefully.

References

1. Ruddick W. Parents and life prospects. In: O'Neill O, Ruddick W, editors. *Having children: philosophical and legal reflections on parenthood.* New York: Oxford University Press; 1979. p. 124.
2. Nelson JL. Taking families seriously. *Hastings Cent Rep* 1992;22(4):6-12.
3. Hardwig J. What about the family? *Hastings Cent Rep* 1990;20(2):5-10.

4. Leikin S. A proposal concerning decisions to forgo life-sustaining treatment for young people. *J Pediatr* 1989;115:17-22.
5. Mahowald M. *Women and children in health care*. New York: Oxford University Press; 1993. p. 187,189.
6. Hellmann J. In pursuit of harmonized values: patient/parent–pediatrician relationships. In: Lynch A, editor. *The "good" pediatrician: an ethics curriculum for use in Canadian pediatrics residency programs*. Toronto: Pediatric Ethics Network; 1996.
7. Pellegrino ED. Toward a reconstruction of medical morality: the primacy of the act of profession and the fact of illness. *J Med Philos* 1979;4(1):31-56.
8. *Malette* v. *Shulman* (1990), 67 DLR (4th) 321 (Ont CA).
9. Art. 11 CCQ.
10. Rozovsky LE, Rozovsky FA. *The Canadian law of consent to treatment*. Toronto: Butterworths; 1992. p. 53-7.
11. *R.B.* v. *Children's Aid Society of Metropolitan Toronto*, [1995] 1 SCR 315.
12. American Academy of Pediatrics. Informed consent, parental permission and assent in pediatric practice. *Pediatrics* 1995;95:314-7.
13. Matthews GR. Children's conceptions of illness and death. In: Kopelman LM, Moskop JC, editors. *Children and health care: moral and social issues*. Dordrecht (Holland): Kluwer Academic Publishers; 1989. p. 133-46.
14. Koocher GP, DeMaso DR. Children's competence to consent to medical procedures. *Pediatrician* 1990;17:68-73.
15. King NMP, Cross AW. Children as decision makers: guidelines for pediatricians. *J Pediatr* 1989;115:10-6.
16. Lewis MA, Lewis CE. Consequences of empowering children to care for themselves. *Pediatrician* 1990;17:63-7.
17. Yoos HL. Children's illness concepts: old and new paradigms. *Pediatr Nurs* 1994;20:134-45.
18. Broome ME, Stieglitz KA. The consent process and children. *Res Nurs Health* 1992;15:147-52.
19. Erlen JA. The child's choice: an essential component in treatment decisions. *Child Health Care* 1987;15:156-60.
20. Baylis F. The moral weight of a child's dissent. *Ethics Med Pract* 1993;3(1):2-3.
21. Weithorn LA, Campbell SB. The competency of children and adolescents to make informed treatment decisions. *Child Dev* 1982;53:1589-98.
22. Lewis CC. How adolescents approach decisions: changes over grades seven to twelve and policy implications. *Child Dev* 1981;52:538-44.
23. Brock DW. Children's competence for health care decisionmaking. In: Kopelman LM, Moskop JC, editors. *Children and health care: moral and social issues*. Dordrecht (Holland): Kluwer Academic Publishers; 1989. p. 181-212.
24. Adams PL, Fras I. *Beginning child psychiatry*. New York: Bruner/Mazel; 1988.
25. Kestenbaum CJ, Williams D, editors. *Handbook of clinical assessment of children and adolescents*. New York: University Press; 1988.
26. Drane JF. The many faces of competency. *Hastings Cent Rep* 1985;15(2):17-21.
27. Freyer DR. Children with cancer: special considerations in the discontinuation of life-sustaining treatment. *Med Pediatr Oncol* 1992;20:136-42.

10

Ethical dilemmas that arise in the care of pregnant women: rethinking "maternal–fetal conflicts"

Elizabeth Flagler, MD; Françoise Baylis, PhD;
Sanda Rodgers, LLB/BCL, LLM

> Ms. X is 19 years old and is 25 weeks pregnant. During a prenatal office visit she reveals that her partner is bisexual and may have been exposed to HIV. Her physician advises her to have an HIV test, explaining that if she is seropositive she can receive treatment that may slow the disease process. Moreover, treatment may reduce the risk of HIV transmission to the fetus. In spite of this information, Ms. X refuses HIV testing.
>
> Ms. Y is 24 years old and has been in labour for 18 hours. The cervical dilatation has not progressed past 3 cm. The fetal heart rate tracing has been worrisome but is now seriously abnormal, showing a profound brady-cardia of 65 beats per minute. This bradycardia does not resolve with con-servative measures. Repeat pelvic examination reveals no prolapsed cord and confirms a vertex presentation at 3 cm dilatation. The obstetrician explains to Ms. Y that cesarean section will be necessary in view of the fetal distress. Ms. Y absolutely refuses, saying "No surgery."

What are maternal–fetal dilemmas?

When a physician believes that he or she has a moral obligation to pursue 2 conflicting courses of action, he or she faces a moral dilemma.[1] In the care of pregnant women, moral dilemmas can arise when the physician believes that the obligation to respect a patient's decision conflicts with the obligation to protect the fetus from harm. This conflict can arise in at least 3 separate realms, that is, with respect to the woman's personal health care choices, lifestyle and behaviours, and occupational situation. In practice and in the literature, these unfortunate situations are often described as "maternal–fetal conflicts."[2–4]

The use of this term is problematic for several reasons. First, it situates the conflict between the pregnant woman and the fetus, whereas the conflict is really between the pregnant woman and others who believe that they know best how to protect the fetus.[5] These others may be seen to act from a sense of professional duty or as agents of the state (on behalf of society at large) and may include third parties such as child welfare agencies, physicians and other health care providers.[3,4,6] Second, the term perpetuates the underlying but unfounded assumption that the problem involves the opposition of maternal rights against fetal rights. At most, there is a conflict between the woman's autonomy and the best interest of the fetus. Some caregivers are committed to respecting the pregnant woman's wishes; others deem that state intervention to protect the fetus is both necessary and appropriate in some circumstances. Finally, the term "maternal–fetal conflict" is factually incorrect. The term "maternal" suggests the existence of parental obligation toward the fetus, whereas the woman is *yet to become* a mother to the fetus she is carrying. This is a significant distinction. Although the term "maternal–fetal conflicts" has gained currency, we advocate the use of the more descriptive phrase, "ethical dilemmas that arise in the care of pregnant women."

Why are ethical dilemmas that arise in the care of pregnant women important?

Ethics

The principle of reproductive freedom stipulates that people have the right to make their own reproductive choices and that the state has an obligation to foster conditions under which this can occur.[7] For some, this principle is morally objectionable because it grants women the right to make decisions concerning the termination of unwanted pregnancies. In their view, whatever rights the pregnant woman may or may not have do not override the fetus' right to life. The problem with this position is that typically it rests on the highly contested premise that the fetus, like the pregnant woman, is a person — someone whose interests and rights must be respected.

Others do not reject the principle of reproductive freedom but at the same time advocate what they believe to be legitimate restrictions on this principle as it applies to women. They maintain that although the fetus may not have the rights of a person, once the woman has decided "of her own free will" to continue the pregnancy she has obligations to the fetus. Moreover, the state may intervene to limit or preclude actions that would irreversibly harm the fetus.[8,9] Again, this position is problematic. It suggests an opposition between the interests of the woman and those of the fetus, and overlooks the important fact that these interests are inextricably linked. The few women who do risk harming their fetuses typically do not actively seek to cause such harm.

All things being equal, women who bring their pregnancy to term do not want damaged babies. But, alas, sometimes a woman's choices are made in ignorance, or are informed by deeply held religious or personal beliefs that preclude certain decisions, or result from strong social and psychological pressures. Any one of these factors can prevent a woman from acting in the best interest of her fetus. Consider, for example, a woman who fears physical and psychological abuse or abandonment by her partner and therefore refuses voluntary HIV testing that might indicate the need for immediate drug therapy to prevent vertical transmission. Were her circumstances different, she would prefer not to have her child born to possibly suffer and die from HIV infection.[10] It should also be noted that continuing a pregnancy does not always involve a deliberate, active choice on the part of the woman. Similarly, many behaviours that may ultimately harm a fetus cannot properly be described as choices, as in the case of addictions.

Recognizing such limitations, some may still argue that state intervention — including forced screening, forced incarceration to prevent continued substance abuse, and forced obstetrical interventions — is morally justified. However, when the issue is considered in its broader social and political context it becomes clear that such interventions are indefensible. First, such coercion is far in excess of any nonvoluntary intervention that would be tolerated to save nonfetal lives. For example, parents are not coerced to become organ donors even when a failure to do so would likely result in the death of their child. We may consider a parent's refusal to make such a donation to be morally reprehensible, but it is beyond the realm of state authority. To coerce a pregnant woman to accept efforts to promote fetal well-being is an unacceptable infringement of her personal autonomy.[11,12]

Second, the harm to women that such coercion represents often occurs without any countervailing benefit to the fetus. For example, there are reports of healthy infants delivered after the woman refused consent for cesarean section that was deemed necessary.[11] Third, state intervention is likely to discourage women whose fetuses may be most at risk from seeking appropriate care.[11,12] It is also likely to undermine the trust between pregnant women and their health care providers that is necessary to foster the education that would promote the birth of healthier babies.

Finally, state intervention to promote fetal well-being is hypocritical given the inconsistency between aggressive efforts made to rescue a few fetuses from a few women in unfortunate situations and the widespread tolerance for unacceptable and sometimes dangerous living conditions in which many children find themselves.

Law

Canadian law addresses 2 issues relevant to this discussion: it confirms the competent woman's right to refuse treatment and the absence of fetal rights. First, informed consent is a legal necessity in medical practice (see chapter 1). Physicians who treat a competent patient without his or her consent put themselves at risk of both criminal and civil liability.[13,14] As well, coercive treatment of a woman by the state contravenes the Canadian Charter of Rights and Freedoms, which recognizes that women and men have equal rights to life, liberty and security of the person.[15]

Second, in common law the fetus does not have legal rights until it is born alive and with complete delivery from the body of the pregnant woman.[16–18] For this reason child protection legislation (which, under certain circumstances, authorizes state intervention) does not apply to the fetus.[19]

A recent decision of the Manitoba Court of Appeal confirms this position.[20] Although the decision of the lower court suggested that there was legal authority to order a pregnant woman to undergo, without consent, counselling and hospital admission to manage a drug addiction, the Court of Appeal confirmed that there was no legal basis on which to do so. This decision confirmed that the fetus is not protected before birth under Canadian law and that the courts have no legal grounds on which to order a competent pregnant woman to undergo a medical intervention that she does not want. An appeal of this case will be heard by the Supreme Court of Canada (see addendum to this chapter).

Policy

The CMA Code of Ethics stipulates that a physician "must respect the right of a competent patient to accept or reject any medical care recommended."[21] Consistent with this position is the recommendation of the Royal College of Physicians and Surgeons of Canada that when a physician's view of the best interest of the fetus conflicts with the view of the pregnant woman, the role of the physician is to provide counselling and persuasion, but not coercion.[22]

This view is discussed more fully in the Final Report of the Royal Commission on New Reproductive Technologies,[23] which recommended that

- medical treatment never be imposed upon a pregnant woman against her wishes,
- criminal law, or any other law, never be used to confine or imprison a pregnant woman in the interest of her fetus,
- the conduct of a pregnant woman in relation to her fetus not be criminalized,

- child welfare or other legislation never be used to control a woman's behaviour during pregnancy, and
- civil liability never be imposed upon a woman for harm done to her fetus during pregnancy.

Empirical studies

One of the justifications for state intervention in pregnancy is the belief that it benefits the fetus. However, reports of good fetal outcomes despite a woman's refusal of cesarean section call this assumption into question.[11,24,25] Unfortunately, there is no standardized system for documenting and assessing cases in which a pregnant woman refuses medical advice.

A review of the few cases that have reached the courts in Canada shows unequivocally that state intervention is disproportionately oppressive of poor women, aboriginal women and women who are members of other racial and ethnic minorities.[26] This finding is cause for concern.

Moreover, the almost exclusive focus on the impact of pregnant women's behaviours and choices on the health and well-being of the fetus reflects an unacceptable gender bias. There is ample evidence to show that paternal drug and alcohol abuse, excessive caffeine and nicotine use, spousal abuse and certain paternal occupations are also potentially hazardous to the fetus.[27–29]

Finally, when attention is directed only toward the pregnant woman's behaviours and choices, the fact that "malnutrition, violence, chaotic lives, serious maternal health problems and lack of medical care"[30] have a significant impact on the health and well-being of the fetus is often overlooked.

How should I approach ethical dilemmas that arise in the care of pregnant women?

Although Canadian law does not recognize fetal rights, fetal interests are taken into consideration by physicians and their pregnant patients. In fact, with the development of detailed ultrasound imaging, excellent perinatal technology and the ability to improve outcomes for very small infants, it is hard for many physicians not to envision the fetus as a patient.[2,31] Thus, some physicians see themselves as having responsibility for 2 "patients" in 1 body. It is extraordinarily difficult for a physician to stand by while a fetus dies or becomes irreparably harmed when an intervention might prevent this result. Nonetheless, it is still inappropriate either to coerce a patient to undergo an intervention or to abandon her.

Difficult as it may be, the physician must respect the competent woman's right to make decisions for herself and her fetus. Moreover, care must be taken not to question the competence of the woman merely because she does not concur with one's recommendations. The most common reason for rejecting medical advice is not incompetence but fear of the unknown. Other possible reasons are denial, past experience, a bias toward the present and near future, and a lack of trust in the medical profession.[32]

Communication, understanding and respect for women are essential in the management of these difficult situations. However, no matter how skilled a communicator the physician might be, a woman may for reasons of her own not alter her decision or behaviour. The physician's communication skills may be significantly tested in such cases (especially when a decision is needed urgently), and it may be difficult to develop the trust that is integral to the physician–patient relationship.

As in other challenging medical situations, consultation with a colleague can be extremely helpful.

Because the treatment of HIV-seropositive pregnant women is believed to benefit the fetus, there is ongoing debate about mandatory HIV testing for pregnant women.[33] However, to respect a pregnant woman's autonomy this intervention may not occur without her explicit consent. Issues of possible prejudice or bias with regard to employment, insurance, housing and so on may factor significantly in decisions about HIV testing. From a practical perspective, it is worth emphasizing that testing alone is not an effective intervention that benefits the fetus. If a woman is found to be HIV seropositive, she has the right to refuse treatment even if such treatment is potentially beneficial to the fetus. Therefore, despite the increased risk that Ms. X may be HIV seropositive, the physician must respect her refusal of HIV testing.

Further discussion clarifies that Ms. Y is terrified of general anesthesia because her mother died from anesthesia complications. Moreover, Ms. Y has a strong distrust of physicians and believes that too many cesarean sections are done. When it is explained that the cesarean can be done with spinal anesthesia, and in view of the risks of the ongoing bradycardia, Ms. Y agrees to the surgery. However, if the patient had continued to refuse the surgery, the physician would have been obliged to respect her decision despite the serious risks to the fetus.

References

1. Beauchamp TL, Childress JF. *Principles of biomedical ethics.* 4th ed. New York: Oxford University Press; 1994. p. 11-3.
2. Steinbock B. Maternal–fetal conflict and in utero fetal therapy. *Albany Law Rev* 1994;57:782-93.
3. Stein EJ. Maternal–fetal conflict: reformulating the equation. In: Grubb A, editor. *Challenges in medical care.* Chichester (England): John Wiley and Sons; 1992. p. 91-2.

4. Mahowald MB. *Women and children in health care: an unequal majority*. New York: Oxford University Press; 1993. p. 131-43.

5. Milliken N. Maternal–fetal relationship. In: Reich WT, editor. *Encyclopedia of bioethics*. Vol 3. New York: Simon and Schuster Macmillan; 1995. p. 406.

6. Nelson LJ. Legal dimensions of maternal–fetal conflict. *Clin Obstet Gynecol* 1992;35(4):738-48.

7. Sherwin S. *No longer patient: feminist ethics and health care*. Philadelphia: Temple University Press; 1992. p. 115-6.

8. Robertson J. Legal issues in prenatal therapy. *Clin Obstet Gynecol* 1986;29(3):603-11.

9. Chervenak FA, McCullogh LB. Perinatal ethics: a practical analysis of obligations to mother and fetus. *Obstet Gynecol* 1985;66:442-6.

10. Kitcher P. *The lives to come: the genetic revolution and human possibilities*. New York: Simon and Schuster; 1996. p. 83.

11. Annas GJ. Protecting the liberty of pregnant patients. *N Engl J Med* 1987;316:1213-4.

12. Mahowald MB. *Women and children in health care: an unequal majority*. New York: Oxford University Press; 1993. p. 143.

13. *Malette* v. *Shulman* (1990), 67 DLR (4th) 321 at 338 (Ont CA).

14. *Criminal Code*, RSC 1985, c C-46.

15. *Canadian Charter of Rights and Freedoms*, s 7, Part I of the *Constitution Act 1982*, being Schedule B to the *Canada Act 1982* (UK), 1982, c 11.

16. *R.* v. *Sullivan* (1988), 65 CR (3d) 256 at 271 (BCCA).

17. Martin S, Coleman M. Judicial intervention in pregnancy. *McGill Law J* 1995:973-80.

18. Rodgers S. Judicial interference with gestation and birth. In: Royal Commission on New Reproductive Technologies. *Legal and ethical issues in new reproductive technologies: pregnancy and parenthood*. vol. 4. Ottawa: Minister of Supply and Services Canada; 1993. p. 457.

19. Knoppers BM, editor. *Canadian child health law*. Toronto: Thompson Educational Publishing; 1992. p. 136.

20. *Winnipeg Child and Family Services (Northwest Area)* v. *D.F.G.* (1996). Reversed on appeal Manitoba Court of Appeal, Sept 12, 1996. Leave to appeal to SCC granted.

21. Canadian Medical Association. Code of ethics. *CMAJ* 1996;155:1176A-B.

22. Cited in *Proceed with care: final report of the Royal Commission on New Reproductive Technologies*. vol 2. Ottawa: Minister of Government Services; 1993. p. 959.

23. *Proceed with care: final report of the Royal Commission on New Reproductive Technologies*. vol. 2. Ottawa: Minister of Government Services; 1993. p. 964-65.

24. Annas GJ. Forced cesareans: the most unkindest cut of all. *Hastings Cent Rep* 1982;12(3):16-7,45.

25. Kolder VEB, Gallagher J, Parsons MT. Court-ordered obstetrical interventions. *N Engl J Med* 1987;316:1192-6.

26. *Proceed with care: final report of the Royal Commission on New Reproductive Technologies*. vol 2. Ottawa: Minister of Government Services; 1993. p. 953.

27. Losco J, Shublack M. Paternal–fetal conflict: an examination of paternal responsibilities to the fetus. *Polit Life Sci* 1994;13(1):63-75.

28. Schroedel JR, Peretz P. A gender analysis of policy formation: the case of fetal abuse. *J Health Polit Policy Law* 1994;19:335-60.

29. Olshan AF, Teschke K, Baird PA. Paternal occupation and congenital anomalies in offspring. *Am J Ind Med* 1991;20:447-75.

30. Pollitt K. "Fetal rights: a new assault on feminism." *Nation* Mar 26, 1990:411.

31. Harrison MR, Golbus MS, Filly RA. *The unborn patient*. New York: Grune and Stratton; 1984.

32. Brock DW, Wartman SA. When competent patients make irrational choices. *N Engl J Med* 1990;322:1595-9.
33. Connor EM, Sperling RS, Gelber R, Kiselev P, Scott G, O'Sullivan MJ, et al, for the Pediatric AIDS Clinical Trials Group Protocol 076 Study Group. Reduction of maternal–infant transmission of human immunodeficiency virus type I with zidovudine treatment. *N Engl J Med* 1994;331:1173-80.

Addendum

In October 1997, the Society of Obstetricians and Gynaecologists of Canada issued a policy statement opposing involuntary intervention in the lives of pregnant women.[1]

On Oct. 31, 1997, the Supreme Court of Canada dismissed the appeal of the Winnipeg Child and Family Services in the Baby G case. Writing the decision for the Supreme Court, Justice McLachlin concluded that "the common law does not clothe the courts with power to order the detention of a pregnant woman for the purpose of preventing harm to her unborn child. Nor, given the magnitude of the changes and their potential ramifications, would it be appropriate for the courts to extend their power to make such an order."[2]

References

1. Involuntary intervention in the lives of pregnant women [policy statement]. *J SOGC* 1997;19(11):1200-3.
2. *Winnipeg Child and Family Services (Northwest Area)* v. *D.F.G.*, [1997] 3 SCR 925.

11

Ethics and genetics in medicine

Michael M. Burgess, PhD; Claude M. Laberge, MD, PhD;
Bartha Maria Knoppers, LLD

Ms. Z is a 25-year-old graduate student. She consults a family physician at the university health clinic because she wants to know if she is a genetic carrier of myotonic dystrophy. Although there is no clinical family history, myotonic dystrophy was recently diagnosed in her older sister after she gave birth to a "floppy" baby. The physician takes a blood sample, sends it to a DNA laboratory for testing and tells her to phone in 3 weeks for the results.

Ms. AA, a 38-year-old woman with 2 teenage daughters, expressed concern to her family physician about her genetic risk for breast cancer. Breast cancer had been diagnosed in her mother when she was 40 years old, and premenopausal ovarian cancer had been diagnosed in her aunt. Ms. AA reports that her sisters, aged 35 and 40 years, are healthy and unconcerned. The family physician refers Ms. AA to the local hereditary cancer program. Ms. AA receives genetic counselling, consents to genetic testing under a research protocol and provides a blood sample. Eighteen months later Ms. AA returns to the family physician on an unrelated matter. She is distraught and tells her family physician that she has the *BRCA1* mutation, is at increased risk of dying in the same awful way that her mother had, and that the genetic counsellor is pressuring her to tell her sisters.

What are the ethics of genetics in medicine?

Molecular genetics is concerned with the process by which the coding sequences of DNA are transcribed into proteins that control cell reproduction, specialization, maintenance and responses. Inherited or acquired biologic factors that result in an error in this molecular information processing can contribute to the development of a disease. Medical genetics involves the application of genetic knowledge and technology to specific clinical and epidemiologic concerns. Although many common diseases are suspected of having a genetic component, few are purely genetic in the sense that the genetic anomaly is adequate to give rise to the disease. In most cases, genetic risk factors must be augmented by other genetic or environmental factors for the disease to be expressed. Moreover, the detection of a genetic anomaly associated with a disorder such as Down's syndrome does not help us to predict the severity with which the syndrome will be expressed.

Predictive testing does exist for a number of monogenic disorders, such as Huntington's disease.[1,2] Genetic testing can be used to confirm a clinical diagnosis, to detect a genetic predisposition to a disease so that preventive measures can be taken or to help a patient prepare for the future, or to give parents the option of terminating a pregnancy or beginning treatment as early as possible.[3] Genetic testing conducted during research contributes to our understanding of the mechanisms of disease and may eventually allow us to identify which subtypes of a syndrome respond well to treatment and which do not. However, the clinical use of genetic testing, which has become common because of its widespread use in research, has been premature. The social and psychosocial implications of genetic information are not well understood, and the development of useful clinical responses to the results of testing has not kept pace with the development of genetic tests.

Certain ethical and legal responsibilities accompany the flood of genetic knowledge into the current practice of medicine. This is because of 3 general characteristics of genetic information: the implications of genetic information are simultaneously individual and familial; genetic information is often relevant to future disease; and genetic testing often identifies disorders for which there are no effective treatments or preventive measures.

Why are the ethics of genetics important in medicine?

Ethics

Although there is no single ethical issue that unifies the field of genetics, informed consent, confidentiality and the potential for social harm and psychological distress are issues that physicians involved with testing should understand. The case examples illustrate the 2 issues, consent to genetic counselling and confidentiality, that family physicians are most likely to be confronted with when managing patients in whom family history or genetic testing may provide valuable genetic information.

Informed consent, which must be obtained before genetic tests are conducted, requires that patients participate in health care decisions. Obtaining informed consent to genetic testing is particularly challenging in view of the complexity of genetic information, the controversial nature of clinical options such as abortion or prophylactic surgery of unknown efficacy, and the social and psychological implications of testing (see chapters 1 and 2). Positive genetic test results are rarely accompanied by the prospect of either treatment or cure. In the absence of effective treatment, the potential for psychological harm and social discrimination must be considered. Patients must evaluate whether the benefit of testing is worth the risk. When genetic testing is part of research, the purpose of the research should be made clear to the patient and uncertainties that might arise as a result of testing discussed (see chapter 12).

Patients have the right to control the use of all medical information about themselves, including genetic information (see chapter 8). The predictive or risk-assessing nature of genetic information makes it valuable to health care planners, insurers and people evaluating long-term concerns such as education, career choices, and risk avoidance and health promotion.[3] The possibility of insurance discrimination has made the confidentiality of genetic information even more important.[4,5] Physicians should ensure that patients understand that after genetic testing their ability to qualify for insurance may be affected. Even though including in clinical records the results of genetic testing conducted in the course of research is not always appropriate,[6] the legal definition of "health care record" includes all written information about a patient. Separate records provide little protection to the patient and may compromise care if the genetic information is such that it would affect treatment in the future or be of interest to a family member. Departments of medical genetics do maintain familial records that link the genetic records of individual patients to assist with the clinical services they provide. Nevertheless, information from these records is typically shared with family members only with the consent of the person whose test results are being disclosed. The familial nature of genetic information can create a conflict for the physician, who has a duty to maintain confidentiality but may feel a duty to warn family members of possible risk. Ultimately, the issues of duty to warn and access to health care records will probably be decided by legislation, whereas consent and access to genetic testing will be evaluated on the basis of social and psychological risk.

Law

Although a ban on germ-line genetic therapy and on prenatal screening for sex selection was proposed as part of the Human Reproductive and Genetic Technologies Act (Bill C-47),[7] currently there is no specific legislation relating to the use of genetic information in Canada. There are 3 main legal issues that apply to clinical genetics: informed consent to testing; standard of care, including genetic counselling for adults and pregnant women wanting to undergo testing; and the duty to warn family members who may be at risk.

There are other legal and ethical issues that are beyond the clinical focus of this chapter. One is whether patent laws that apply to genetic research serve the public interest.[8] A second is whether legislation should protect people from the use of genetic tests as a basis for discrimination by employers and insurers.

Explicit informed consent to a genetic test is required because genetic testing carries considerable risk of social harm in the form of discrimination. A patient might reasonably consider that the possibility of discrimination would outweigh the benefits of the test, particularly if no effective treatment or preventive measures are available.

There is no standard of care for clinical genetic practice, and the test and counselling programs that are offered vary among provinces. However, current case law indicates that physicians have a legal obligation to inform patients of the availability of prenatal testing.[9–11] Generally, geneticists suggest that obstetricians offer prenatal tests when the risk of a serious genetic condition outweighs the risk of spontaneous miscarriage caused by amniocentesis or chorionic villae sampling. Much genetic testing is conducted as research, and aspects of a study design, such as the use of cloning or the objective of gene therapy, may be relevant to physicians or patients. Ethical concerns specific to genetic research are beyond the scope of this chapter and are discussed in chapter 12 and elsewhere.[6,12,13]

The duty to warn family members about a genetic condition is based on the premise that the warning is necessary to avert serious harm. As discussed in chapter 8, any breach of confidentiality must be based on a realistic assessment of whether the disclosure will effectively prevent serious harm. This breach of confidentiality is rarely justified, except in cases where prevention or treatment is possible, such as for familial adenomatous polyposis.[14–16] A physician contemplating warning a family member about a genetic risk should be able to answer "yes" to the following questions:

- Is the family member at a high risk of serious harm?
- Does the breach of confidentiality actually make it possible to prevent or minimize the harm?
- Is the breach of confidentiality necessary to prevent or minimize the harm (i.e., has the patient refused to disclose the information or to give consent for its disclosure).

Policy

Policy guidelines and recommendations are often established for specific diseases with genetic components. The most common theme of such guidelines is the requirement for pre- and post-test genetic counselling. The importance of having a competent professional provide the counselling has been noted, but there are not enough specifically trained genetic counsellors or clinical geneticists to handle the anticipated caseload as genetic testing becomes more common.[17,18] There is general agreement that health care professionals who provide genetic counselling must be well informed about the nature of the condition and the social and psychological implications of genetic testing, and must be able to interpret the test results and assess specific familial genetic risks.[19–23]

Empirical studies

Much of the empirical work in genetics and ethics has related to studies of knowledge of genetics, attitudes toward testing and the psychological effects of available genetic tests. These studies have shown that among Canadian health care professionals, understanding of genetics is poor[17] and there is wide practice variation with respect to genetic testing.[18] Most research into specific diseases suggests that when it is accompanied by adequate counselling, genetic testing is safe and beneficial, even when effective treatments or preventive measures are not available. For example, studies of predictive testing for Huntington's disease found that the psychological well-being of patients improved after testing, and few of the suicidal and depressive episodes that were anticipated actually occurred.[23–25] Despite an emphasis on a nondirective presentation of all options in genetic counselling, studies have found that the subtle influence of counsellors' values may affect patients' choices.[26–29] Psychologists and members of families at risk have pushed for research that is more process- and family-oriented,[30,31] and new studies have tried to determine the effect genetic knowledge has on self-concept and family relationships. Some studies even suggest that the most significant and ethically relevant effects of genetic testing may be on the relationship between the health care provider and the patient and among family members.[32–35]

How should I approach ethics and genetics in practice?

Media coverage and the very significant investment being made in genetic research will likely increase the number of patients who want to discuss genetic risk and testing with their family physicians. It is not appropriate to simply order genetic tests and then deal with the results and implications if the test result is "positive." Consent and confidentiality require a thorough discussion and realistic planning before the test is conducted.

Genetic counselling has been developed to manage the delivery of complex information and the moral controversies surrounding such issues as abortion and lifestyle changes. It also meets the ethical requirement of informed consent and provides support for patients facing testing. Counselling involves a detailed disclosure and supportive discussion designed to help patients understand these issues as well as those related to genetic research and duties to family members (e.g., banking of tissue samples for future DNA testing, the social risks and obligations of patients to family members that may affect confidentiality).[13,36,37] Counselling should also clearly establish that there is a possibility that paternity might become an issue, but this is not typically included in the information disclosed. Genetic counselling includes following up with patients to ensure that they have been able to integrate test results and their implications into their lives. One of the primary purposes of the testing is to help patients plan for the future. However, genetic counsellors and geneticists cannot always anticipate or understand how familial and social influences will affect the way a patient responds to and uses genetic information.[26,32,33,38]

As with all medical information, genetic information should not be disclosed to third parties or family members without the patient's consent. The exceptions are those rare cases where treatment or preventive measures are available and family members are unaware they are at risk.[14–16] People buying insurance are frequently required to divulge all risk information and to sign a release form that gives the insurance company access to their health care records, which may include genetic test results (whether clinical or research).[4,5] Concealing genetic test results from an insurance company may nullify a policy, which could negatively affect a person's future health care. When appropriate, the options for DNA banking, including current or future access by family members or researchers should be discussed with the patient.[37] Family physicians and specialists must share the burden of integrating genetic information into the health care system. However, physicians may find that requests related to specific diseases may be too infrequent to justify investing time and resources in learning about them. Physicians who have patients interested in genetic testing will have to evaluate whether to refer those patients to genetic centres or to take on the responsibility of genetic counselling themselves.

Ms. Z received genetic testing without adequate counselling. In such situations the informed consent may be invalid and the patient may not be adequately prepared for the information the genetic test provides. Results should be delivered in a supportive manner so the patient understands the implications of the test information and can begin to work through the accompanying risks and responsibilities. Delivering the results over the phone is not supportive. In order to counsel a patient, the physician must know and communicate the risk of being a carrier, which can be as high as 50%. The physician should have asked Ms. Z why she wanted to know her status to determine whether she understood the purpose of genetic testing and whether genetic testing would meet her needs.

The family physician referred Ms. AA to a local hereditary cancer program for counselling and testing. Most genetic counselling programs include a discussion about the need to talk to family members about genetic risks. For genetic testing to be included in a research protocol, counselling would likely be mandated by a research ethics board.[13] The issue that remains is how the family physician can help the woman deal with her test results, including whether and what to tell her sisters. Any breach of confidentiality on the part of the physician must be justified by the risk of serious harm and the benefits of disclosure. The sisters could be told that they have a 50% chance of having a mutation that would significantly increase the risk of breast or ovarian cancer developing before age 65. The physician has no way of knowing how the sisters would react to this information but must assess how useful it would be to them. There is no guaranteed prophylaxis for breast cancer, but early detection and treatment may lead to a better outcome. There are social and psychological risks associated with informing and not informing the sisters. At this time, the speculative nature of the benefits of knowing they are at increased risk does not support a legal duty to warn the sisters, although it may be ethically permissible.[18] To respect Ms. AA's confidentiality, however, the physician should continue to encourage her to discuss the genetic risks with her sisters.

References

1. Huntington's Disease Collaborative Research Group. A novel gene containing a trinucleotide repeat that is expanded and unstable in Huntington's disease chromosomes. *Cell* 1993;72:971-83.
2. Kremer B, Goldberg P, Andrew SE, Squitieri F, Theilmann J, Telenius H, et al, and the International Huntington Disease Research Group. World-wide study of the Huntington's disease mutation: the sensitivity and specificity of repeated CAG sequences. *N Engl J Med* 1994;330:1401-6.
3. Lemmens T. "What about your genes?" Ethical, legal and policy dimensions of genetics in the workplace. *Politics Life Sci* 1997;16(1):57-75.
4. Lemmens T, Bahamin P. Genetics in life, disability and additional health insurance in Canada: a legal and ethical analysis. Report to Medical, Ethical, Legal and Social Issues Advisory Committee of Canadian Genome Analysis and Technology Programme, 1996 Nov.
5. NIH-DOE Working Group on Ethical, Legal, and Social Implications of Human Genome Research. *Genetic information and health insurance.* Report of the Task Force. Bethesda (MD): National Institutes of Health; 1993.
6. Glass KC, Weijer C, Lemmens T, Palmour R, Shapiro SH. Structuring the review of human genetics protocols. Part II: diagnostic and screening studies. *IRB: Rev Hum Subj Res* 1997;19(3.4):1-11,13.

7. Bill C-47, *An Act respecting human reproductive technologies and commercial transactions relating to human reproduction*. 2d sess, 35th Parl, 1996.
8. Caulfield T, Hirtle M, Le Bris S. Regulating NRTs in Canada: Is commercialization the solution for Canada? *Health Law Can* 1997;18:3-14.
9. *H(R)* v. *Hunter* (1996), 32 CCLT (2d) 44 (Ont Ct [Gen Div]).
10. *Arndt* v. *Smith* (1997), 148 DLR (4th) 48 (SCC).
11. Caulfield T, Robertson G. Eugenic policies in Alberta: From the systematic to the systemic? *Alta Law Rev* 1996;35:59-79.
12. Glass KC, Weijer C, Palmour R, Shapiro SH, Lemmens T, Lebacqz K. Structuring the review of human genetics protocols: gene localization and identification studies. *IRB: Rev Hum Subj Res* 1996;18(4):1-9.
13. Medical Research Council of Canada, Natural Sciences and Engineering Research Council of Canada, Social Sciences and Humanities Research Council of Canada. *Tri-Council policy statement: ethical conduct for research involving humans*. Ottawa: The Councils; 1998. Available: www.mrc.gc.ca and www.sshrc.ca
14. Ontario's Medical Expert Panel on the Duty to Inform. *Final recommendations*. Toronto: Institute for Clinical Evaluative Sciences in Ontario; 1996:A285-97.
15. *Duty to warn: report from council members' dialogue*. Toronto: College of Physicians and Surgeons of Ontario; 1996. p. 21-2.
16. American Society of Human Genetics Social Issues Committee. Points to consider: professional duty to inform of familial genetic information. *Am J Hum Genet* 1998;62:474-83.
17. Wertz DC. Professional perspectives: a survey of Canadian providers. In: Professional norms in the practice of human genetics [special edition]. *Health Law J* 1995;3:59-130.
18. Laberge CM, Knoppers BM, Panisset I. Multidisciplinary perceptions of human genetics in Canada: "Delphi" results with regards to the practice of medical genetics. In: Professional norms in the practice of human genetics [special]. *Health Law J* 1995;3:19-57.
19. Knoppers BM, Caulfield T, Kinsella DT, editors. *Legal rights and human genetic material*. Toronto: Emond Montgomery Publications; 1996.
20. Royal Commission on New Reproductive Technologies. *Proceed with care: final report*. Ottawa: Minister of Public Works; 1993.
21. Knoppers BM. *Human dignity and genetic heritage*. Ottawa: Law Reform Commission of Canada; 1991.
22. Science Council of Canada. *Genetics in Canadian health care*. Ottawa: Minister for Science; 1991.
23. Ontario Law Reform Commission. *Report on genetic testing*. Toronto: The Commission; 1996.
24. Benjami CM, Adam S, Wiggins S, Theilmann JL, Copley TT, Bloch M, et al, and the Canadian Collaborative Groups for Predictive Testing for Huntington Disease. Proceed with care: direct predictive testing for Huntington disease. *Am J Hum Genet* 1994;55:606-17.
25. Codori AM, Brandt J. Psychological costs and benefits of predictive testing for Huntington's disease. *Am J Med Genet* 1994;54:174-84.
26. Rapp R. Chromosomes and communication: the discourse of genetic counselling. *Med Anthropol Q* 1988;2:143-57.
27. Lippman A. Prenatal diagnosis: Reproductive choice? Reproductive control? In: Overall C, editor. *The future of human reproduction*. Toronto: The Women's Press; 1989. p. 182-94.

28. Rothman BK. *The tentative pregnancy.* New York: Viking Press; 1986.
29. Kolker A, Burke M. *Prenatal testing: a sociological perspective.* London: Bergin & Garvey; 1994. p. 31-45.
30. Hayes CV. Genetic testing for Huntington's disease — a family issue [editorial comment]. *N Engl J Med* 1992;327:1449-51.
31. Kessler S, Bloch M. Social system responses to Huntington disease. *Fam Process* 1989;28:59-68.
32. Richards MPM. The new genetics: some issues for social scientists. *Soc Health Illness* 1993;15:567-86.
33. van der Steenstraten IM, Tibben A, Roos RA, van de Kamp JJ, Niermeijer MF. Predictive testing for Huntington disease: non-participants compared with participants in the Dutch program. *Am J Hum Genet* 1994;55:618-25.
34. Quaid K, Wesson MK. Exploration of the effects of predictive testing for Huntington disease on intimate relationships. *Am J Med Genet* 1995;57:46-51.
35. Burgess MM. Ethical issues in genetic testing of Alzheimer disease. *Alzheimer Dis Assoc Disord* 1994;9:71-8.
36. Knoppers BM, Laberge C. DNA sampling and informed consent. *CMAJ* 1989;140:1023-8.
37. Knoppers BM, Laberge CM. Research and stored tissues: persons as sources, samples as persons? [editorial] *JAMA* 1995;274:1806-7.
38. Burgess MM, Hayden MR. Patients' rights to laboratory data: trinucleotide repeat length in Huntington disease [editorial]. *Am J Med Genet* 1996;62:6-9.

12

Research ethics

Charles Weijer, MD, PhD; Bernard M. Dickens, PhD, LLD;
Eric M. Meslin, PhD

> Dr. BB is a family practitioner with a special interest in the treatment of HIV infection and AIDS. He receives a letter from the coordinator of a study to evaluate a promising new treatment for the prevention of HIV-related dementia. The letter invites Dr. BB to submit the names of potentially eligible patients. He will be paid $100 for each name provided.
>
> Dr. CC, a psychiatrist in private practice, is approached by a pharmaceutical company to assist with a clinical trial to test the efficacy of a new drug in the treatment of acute psychosis. The study will enrol acutely psychotic patients with no history of psychosis (or of treatment with antipsychotic drugs) through physicians' offices and emergency departments. Patients enrolled in the study will be randomly assigned to receive the new medication or a placebo and will remain in hospital for 8 weeks. During this time they will not be permitted to receive antipsychotic medications other than the study drug. Informed consent will be obtained from each participant or a proxy. Patients may be withdrawn from the study if their medical condition worsens substantially.

What is research ethics?

Research involving human subjects can raise difficult and important ethical and legal questions. The field of research ethics is devoted to the systematic analysis of such questions to ensure that study participants are protected and, ultimately, that clinical research is conducted in a way that serves the needs of such participants and of society as a whole.

Why is research ethics important?

Many of the ethical issues that arise in human experimentation — such as those surrounding informed consent, confidentiality and the physician's duty of care to the patient — overlap with ethical issues in clinical practice. Nevertheless, important differences exist between research activities and clinical practice. In clinical practice, the physician has a clear obligation to the patient; in research, this obligation remains but may come into conflict with other obligations — and incentives.[1] The researcher has an obligation to ensure that the study findings are valid and replicable, and this has implications for the design and execution of the study. For example, the study must be designed in such a way that the research question can be answered reliably and efficiently; sufficient numbers of patients must be enrolled in a reasonable period; and study participants must comply with their allocated treatment. Substantial rewards can accrue to the successful completion of a research project, such as renewed funding, academic promotion, salary increases, respect from colleagues and, in some cases, fame. Unfortunately, in a number of research studies, including some conducted in Canada, the welfare of individual patients has been sacrificed to these competing interests.[2,3] Various ethical principles, legal requirements and policy statements have been formulated in an attempt to ensure that clinical research is conducted in accordance with the highest scientific and ethical standards.

Ethics

The predominant ethical framework for human experimentation was set out by the US National Commission for the Protection of Human Subjects of Biomedical and Behavioral Research in the Belmont Report.[4] This report articulated 3 guiding principles for research: respect for persons, beneficence and justice. Respect for persons requires that the choices of autonomous individuals be respected and that people who are incapable of making their own choices be protected. This principle underlies the requirement to obtain informed consent from study participants and to maintain confidentiality on their behalf.[5] The principle of beneficence requires that participation in research be associated with a favourable balance of potential benefits and harms.[6] The principle of justice entails an equitable distribution of the burdens and benefits of research. Researchers must not exploit vulnerable people or exclude without good reason eligible candidates who may benefit from participation in a study.[7]

The principles set out in the Belmont Report do not, however, exhaust the ethical requirements for clinical research.[8] Conditions such as the following must also be met.

- A study must employ a *scientifically valid design* to answer the research question. Shoddy science is never ethical.[9,10]
- A study must address a *question of sufficient value* to justify the risk posed to participants. Exposing subjects even to low risk to answer a trivial question is unacceptable.[9]
- A study must be *conducted honestly*. It should be carried out as stated in the approved protocol, and research ethics boards have an obligation to ensure that this is the case.[11]
- Study findings must be *reported accurately and promptly*. Methods, results and conclusions must be reported completely and without exaggeration to allow practising clinicians to draw reasonable conclusions.[12,13] Whenever possible, study results should be reported quickly to allow physicians timely access to potentially important clinical information.[14]

Law

The researcher's duty to have informed consent from research subjects is established in law. The legal doctrine often described as "informed consent" is better understood as "informed choice," since a physician's legal duty is to inform the patient so that he or she may exercise *choice* — which does not always result in *consent*. The physician's duty to disclose information relevant to the choice that the patient is asked to make falls under an aspect of civil law: the law of negligence. A physician may be found negligent if a patient's choice (including the choice to forgo treatment) is inadequately informed and results in harm.[15] Accordingly, patients who are invited to enter a study must be informed of, among other things, the nature and extent of the known risks of participation, the possibility that participation may present unknown risks, and the intended benefit of the study to participants and others. A subject's treatment in a trial without consent may be grounds for legal action on the basis of "unauthorized touching," which is dealt with in 2 domains: assault in criminal law and battery in civil law.

The duty to ensure confidentiality is founded in the physician–patient contract, fiduciary duty and legislation. Confidentiality is a usually implicit term of the physician–patient contract (that is, the tacit agreement between physician and patient on the rendering of care), and its violation is therefore a basis for legal action against the physician. Increasingly, however, as physicians move from fee-for-service payment to salaries or other remuneration systems, confidentiality is addressed under the law of fiduciary duty.[16] Fiduciary duty — the highest standard of duty implied by law — requires that physicians disclose information about a patient only in the patient's best interests and that they avoid any conflict of interest in the disclosure of patient information (even if that information is contained in records physicians lawfully hold). Unauthorized disclosure is actionable as a breach of fiduciary duty. It may also violate a duty of confidentiality enacted in provincial legislation (which varies substantially from province to province). For example, the Civil Code of Quebec is so protective of patient information that anonymous epidemiologic studies may be unlawful without the consent of each person whose medical record is used.[17]

Policy

A number of international policies guide the conduct of research. Although the Nuremberg Code and the International Covenant on Civil and Political Rights remain important early statements,[18,19] the World Medical Association's Declaration of Helsinki, as amended most recently in October 1996, is probably the most influential document governing research world wide.[12] Many of the requirements set out under "Ethics" in this article reflect the Declaration of Helsinki. The Declaration highlights an important additional requirement: patients' participation in research should not put them at a disadvantage with respect to medical care.

Canadian researchers conducting studies funded by the US National Institutes of Health must do so in accordance with the regulations of the US Department of Health and Human Services.[20] Researchers conducting research in other countries should consult the guidelines of the Council for International Organizations of Medical Sciences.[21,22] Geneticists should consult the guidelines developed by the Human Genome Organization.[23]

Medical research in Canada, including studies conducted in the drug approval process, is governed by guidelines of the Medical Research Council (MRC) of Canada.[24,25] These guidelines define research as "the generation of data about persons, through intervention or otherwise, that goes beyond that necessary for the individual person's immediate well being."[24] Proposals for research involving human subjects must be submitted to a local research ethics board for review. Research that will not generate generalizable knowledge (e.g., quality assurance research for internal use and not intended for publication) is generally considered exempt from such review.

The Tri-Council Working Group, a collaboration of the MRC, the Natural Sciences and Engineering Research Council of Canada and the Social Sciences and Humanities Research Council of Canada, is preparing the final version of its code of conduct for research involving humans. A draft document, released in March 1996, generated considerable interest and controversy.[26] It proposed important new standards with respect to research involving communities or "collectivities" (including a requirement to involve community members, where appropriate, in the design process) and the inclusion of women (including "potentially pregnant" and pregnant women) in clinical studies. It also proposed the clear prohibition of placebo-controlled studies when effective standard treatment exists. If the final version closely resembles the draft document in these respects, substantial changes in the conduct of research in Canada will ensue.

Empirical studies

Empirical studies have much to contribute to our understanding of informed consent and the risks and benefits of participation in research. For example, if the principle of respect for persons is to be upheld, it follows that research subjects must not only be *informed* of the purpose, nature, risks, benefits and alternatives associated with their participation but must also *understand* this information. But how well *do* research subjects understand information presented to them in the consent process? The answer seems to be "not well at all."[27] Indeed, because of a phenomenon that Appelbaum and colleagues[28] refer to as "therapeutic misconception," patients commonly believe that experimental projects are tailored to optimize their individual care. In its final report, the White House Advisory Committee on Human Radiation Experiments detailed the results of a survey of 1900 research participants and concluded that serious deficiencies remain in the current system of protecting human subjects of research.[29]

Two lessons follow from the empirical studies on informed consent to participation in research. First, researchers need to establish and maintain effective strategies to ensure that research subjects comprehend the information they are given during the consent process. In an elegant review of this topic, Silva and Sorrell list a wide range of methods available to improve participants' understanding.[30] Second, although such additional measures are important, the empirical data highlight the inadequacy of consent alone to protect study participants. Consent is an important component of this protection, but a research study must present an acceptable balance of risks and benefits as well.[31]

Empirical studies on the risks and benefits of research participation have also made an important contribution to research ethics. For many years, participation in research was viewed as a risky endeavour, one from which people ought to be protected.[32] However, a number of studies in the late 1970s and early 1980s showed that the risks associated with study participation were, in reality, relatively small.[33] Indeed, recent empirical work in oncology suggests that cancer patients who participated in clinical trials received — apart from the specific study treatment — a *net benefit*, namely, improved survival.[34-37] If further study establishes conclusively that trial participation *in itself* is associated with a higher probability of benefit, it may be that prospective study participants should be informed of this fact.

How should I approach research ethics in practice?

Ethical issues in research must not be addressed by researchers as an afterthought. Ethical issues permeate research and must guide research design. What should be used as a control treatment? Who should be included or excluded from a study? How large should the sample be? All of these questions have an ethical component.[38] Researchers ought, therefore, to consider ethical issues from the first stages of planning.

What resources are available to researchers to guide them in ethical matters? Clearly, all Canadian physicians involved in research ought to be familiar with the key documents outlined earlier, particularly the Tri-Council guidelines. Though directed primarily toward an American audience, a number of excellent reference texts are available.[5,39] To our knowledge, the only peer-reviewed journal devoted exclusively to research ethics is *IRB: A Review of Human Subjects Research* — an excellent source for the researcher in an ethical quandary. Finally, and perhaps most important, clinicians should routinely consult with colleagues who have expertise in the ethics of research, including members of research ethics boards.

Dr. BB is offered a financial reward if he will provide the names of patients to a third party who is coordinating a research study. Such "finders' fees" are ethically and legally objectionable.[40] Physicians act in breach of fiduciary duty and in conflict of interest if they use their professional knowledge of a patient's medical or other circumstances for their personal benefit. First, names may not be given to third parties without patient consent. A physician who believes that entry into a study may benefit an eligible patient should inform that patient and let the patient decide whether his or her name may be given to the investigator. Second, physicians must not accept a fee based on the number of names provided. If a physician is asked to consult patients' records or to do other searches, he or she may be remunerated for the time required to perform that service, whether or not any patients are identified and consent to participate.

Dr. CC is invited to enrol his patients in a placebo-controlled study of a new antipsychotic drug. Is it ethical for him to recommend the study to his patients? No. As we have discussed, consent alone is an insufficient ethical basis for enrolling patients in a study: the study must present a favourable balance of benefits and harms. A physician may recommend participation in a study only if the treatments being studied are in a state of "clinical equipoise," that is, if there is "genuine uncertainty" within "the expert clinical community about the comparative merits of the alternatives to be tested."[41] In other words, genuine uncertainty must exist in the community of expert practitioners as to the preferred treatment.[41] When effective standard treatment exists for a disease, as it does for schizophrenia,[42] it is unethical (since placebo is an inferior "treatment") to expose patients to the risk of "treatment" with placebo alone. Practising physicians may be told that placebo controls are necessary in clinical research for scientific, ethical or regulatory reasons. Freedman and colleagues have reviewed these claims comprehensively and conclude that practitioners should regard them with scepticism.[43,44]

References

1. Hellman S, Hellman D. Of mice but not men: problems of the randomized clinical trial. *N Engl J Med* 1991;324:1584-9.
2. Weijer C. The breast cancer research scandal: addressing the issues. *CMAJ* 1995;152:1195-7.
3. Elliott C, Weijer C. Cruel and unusual treatment. *Saturday Night* 1995;110(10):31-4.
4. National Commission for the Protection of Human Subjects of Biomedical and Behavioral Research. The Belmont Report: ethical principles and guidelines for the protection of human subjects of research. *OPRR [Office for Protection from Research Risks] Reports* 1979(Apr 18):1-8.
5. Levine RJ. *Ethics and regulation of clinical research*. New Haven (CT): Yale University Press; 1988:95-153.
6. Levine RJ. *Ethics and regulation of clinical research*. New Haven (CT): Yale University Press; 1988. p. 37-65.
7. Levine RJ. *Ethics and regulation of clinical research*. New Haven (CT): Yale University Press; 1988. p. 67-93.
8. Meslin EM, Sutherland HJ, Lavery JV, Till JE. Principlism and the ethical appraisal of clinical trials. *Bioethics* 1995;9:399-418.
9. Freedman B. Scientific value and validity as ethical requirements for research: a proposed explanation. *IRB: Rev Hum Subj Res* 1987;17(6):7-10.
10. Sutherland HJ, Meslin EM, Till JE. What's missing from current clinical trials guidelines? A framework for integrating science, ethics and the community. *J Clin Ethics* 1994;5:297-303.
11. Weijer C, Shapiro S, Fuks A, Glass KC, Skrutkowska M. Monitoring clinical research: an obligation unfulfilled. *CMAJ* 1995;152:1973-80.
12. World Medical Association. Declaration of Helsinki [1964, rev 1975, 1983, 1989]. In: Reich WT, editor. *Encyclopedia of bioethics*. rev ed. New York: Simon & Schuster Macmillan; 1995. p. 2765-7.
13. International Committee of Medical Journal Editors. Uniform requirements for manuscripts submitted to biomedical journals. *CMAJ* 1997;156:270-7.
14. Meslin EM. Toward an ethic in dissemination of new knowledge in primary care research. In: Dunn EV, editor. *Disseminating research/changing practice: research methods for primary care*. vol 6. Thousand Oaks (CA): Sage Publications; 1994. p. 32-44.
15. *Truman* v. *Thomas*, 611 P 2d 902 (Cal Sup Ct 1980).
16. Dickens BM. Medical records — patient's right to receive copies — physician's fiduciary duty of disclosure: *McInerney* v. *MacDonald*. *Can Bar Rev* 1994;73:234-42.
17. Deleury E, Croubau D. *Le droit des personnes physiques*. Cowansville (QC): Éditions Yvon Blais; 1994. p. 119-20.

18. Nuremberg Code [1947]. In: Reich WT, editor. *Encyclopedia of bioethics.* rev ed. New York: Simon & Schuster Macmillan; 1995. p. 2763-4.

19. General Assembly of the United Nations: International covenant on civil and political rights [1958]. In: Reich WT, editor. *Encyclopedia of bioethics.* rev ed. New York: Simon & Schuster Macmillan; 1995. p. 2765.

20. US Department of Health and Human Services. *Protection of human subjects* [part 46 of *Code of federal regulations,* title 45 (*Public welfare*)]. rev 1991 June 18. Washington: The Department; 1991.

21. Council for International Organizations of Medical Sciences. *International ethical guidelines for biomedical research involving human subjects.* Geneva: The Council; 1993.

22. Council for International Organizations of Medical Sciences. *International guidelines for ethical review of epidemiological studies.* Geneva: The Council; 1991.

23. Human Genome Organization. Statement on the principled conduct of genetic research. *Genome Digest* 1996;3(2):2-3.

24. *Guidelines on research involving human subjects.* Ottawa: Medical Research Council of Canada; 1987.

25. *Drugs directorate guidelines: conduct of clinical investigations.* Ottawa: Health Protection Branch, Health Canada; 1989.

26. Tri-Council Working Group. *Code of conduct for research involving humans* [draft document]. Ottawa: Department of Supply and Services; 1996.

27. Riecken HW, Ravich R. Informed consent to biomedical research in Veterans Administration Hospitals. *JAMA* 1982;248:344-8.

28. Appelbaum PS, Roth LH, Lidz CW, Benson P, Winslade W. False hopes and best data: consent to research and the therapeutic misconception. *Hastings Cent Rep* 1987;17(2):20-4.

29. White House Advisory Committee on Human Radiation Experiments. *Final report* [doc no 061-000-00-848-9]. Washington: The Committee; 1995.

30. Silva MC, Sorrell JM. Enhancing comprehension of information for informed consent: a review of empirical research. *IRB: Rev Hum Subj Res* 1988;10(1):1-5.

31. US Department of Health and Human Services. *Protection of human subjects* [part 46 of *Code of federal regulations,* title 45 (*Public welfare*)]. rev 1991 June 18. Washington: The Department; 1991. p. 111(a).

32. Levine RJ. The impact of HIV infection on society's perception of clinical trials. *Kennedy Inst Ethics J* 1994;4:93-8.

33. Weijer C. Evolving ethical issues in selection of subjects for clinical research. *Camb Q Health Ethics* 1996;5:334-45.

34. Boros L, Chuange C, Butler FO, Bennett JM. Leukemia in Rochester: a 17-year experience with an analysis of the role of cooperative group (ECOG [Eastern Cooperative Oncology Group]) participation. *Cancer* 1985;56:2161-9.

35. Karjalainen S, Palva I. Do treatment protocols improve end results? A study of the survival of patients with multiple myeloma in Finland. *BMJ* 1989;299:1069-72.

36. Hjorth M, Holmberg E, Rodjer S, Westin J. Impact of active and passive exclusions on the results of a clinical trial in multiple myeloma. *Br J Haematol* 1992;80:55-61.

37. Weijer C, Freedman B, Fuks A, Robbins J, Shapiro S, Skrutkowska M. What difference does it make to be treated in a clinical trial? A pilot study. *Clin Invest Med* 1996;19:179-83.

38. Freedman B. Shapiro S. Ethics and statistics in clinical research: towards a more comprehensive examination. *J Stat Plann Inference* 1994;42:223-40.

39. Office for Protection from Research Risk. *Protecting human subjects: institutional review board guidebook.* Washington: The Office; 1993.

40. Lind SE. Finder's fees for research subjects. *N Engl J Med* 1990;323:192-5.
41. Freedman B. Equipoise and the ethics of clinical research. *N Engl J Med* 1987;317:141-5.
42. Kane JM. Schizophrenia. *N Engl J Med* 1996;334:34-41.
43. Freedman B, Weijer C, Glass KC. Placebo orthodoxy in clinical research. I: Empirical and methodological myths. *J Law Med Ethics* 1996;24:243-51.
44. Freedman B, Glass KC, Weijer C. Placebo orthodoxy in clinical research. II: Ethical, legal and regulatory myths. *J Law Med Ethics* 1996;24:252-9.

Authors' note: Dr. Weijer's research is funded by an Operating Grant and Scholar Award from the Medical Research Council of Canada.
Editor's note: The Tri-Council policy statement, *Ethical conduct for research involving humans,* was released on Sept. 17, 1998. This is the definitive research ethics document in Canada at this time. The full text is available on the Web sites of the MRC (www.mrc.gc.ca) and the Social Sciences and Humanities Research Council of Canada (www.sshrc.ca).

13

Euthanasia and assisted suicide

James V. Lavery, MSc; Bernard M. Dickens, PhD, LLD;
Joseph M. Boyle, PhD; Peter A. Singer, MD, MPH

Ms. DD is 32 years old and has advanced gastric cancer that has resulted in constant severe pain and poorly controlled vomiting. Despite steady increases in her morphine dose, her pain has worsened greatly over the last 2 days. Death is imminent, but the patient pleads incessantly with the hospital staff to "put her out of her misery."

Mr. EE is a 39-year-old injection drug user with a history of alcoholism and depression. He presents at an emergency department, insisting that he no longer wishes to live. He repeatedly requests euthanasia on the grounds that he is no longer able to bear his suffering (although he is not in any physical pain). A psychiatrist rules out clinical depression.

What are euthanasia and assisted suicide?

A special Senate committee appointed to inform the national debate on euthanasia and assisted suicide defined euthanasia as "a deliberate act undertaken by one person with the intention of ending the life of another person to relieve that person's suffering where the act is the cause of death."[1] Euthanasia may be "voluntary," "involuntary" or "nonvoluntary," depending on (a) the competence of the recipient, (b) whether or not the act is consistent with his or her wishes (if these are known) and (c) whether or not the recipient is aware that euthanasia is to be performed.

Assisted suicide was defined by the Senate committee as "the act of intentionally killing oneself with the assistance of another who deliberately provides the knowledge, means, or both."[1] In "physician-assisted suicide" a physician provides the assistance.

Why are euthanasia and assisted suicide important?

There is increasing pressure to resolve the question of whether physicians and other health care professionals should in certain circumstances participate in intentionally bringing about the death of a patient and whether these practices should be accepted by society as a whole. The ethical, legal and public-policy implications of these questions merit careful consideration.

Ethics

There is considerable disagreement about whether euthanasia and assisted suicide are ethically distinct from decisions to forgo life-sustaining treatments.[2–10] At the heart of the debate is the ethical significance given to the intentions of those performing these acts.[11,12] Supporters of euthanasia and assisted suicide reject the argument that there is an ethical distinction between these acts and acts of forgoing life-sustaining treatment. They claim, instead, that euthanasia and assisted suicide are consistent with the right of patients to make autonomous choices about the time and manner of their own death.[2,13]

Opponents of euthanasia and assisted suicide claim that death is a predictable consequence of the morally justified withdrawal of life-sustaining treatments only in cases where there is a fatal underlying condition, and that it is the condition, not the action of withdrawing treatment, that causes death.[14] A physician who performs euthanasia or assists in a suicide, on the other hand, has the death of the patient as his or her primary objective.

Although opponents of euthanasia and assisted suicide recognize the importance of self-determination, they argue that individual autonomy has limits and that the right to self-determination should not be given ultimate standing in social policy regarding euthanasia and assisted suicide.[15]

Supporters of euthanasia and assisted suicide believe that these acts benefit terminally ill patients by relieving their suffering,[16] whereas opponents argue that the compassionate grounds for endorsing these acts cannot ensure that euthanasia will be limited to people who request it voluntarily.[17] Opponents of euthanasia are also concerned that the acceptance of euthanasia may contribute to an increasingly casual attitude toward private killing in society.[18]

Most commentators make no formal ethical distinction between euthanasia and assisted suicide, since in both cases the person performing the euthanasia or assisting the suicide deliberately facilitates the patient's death. Concerns have been expressed, however, about the risk of error, coercion or abuse that could arise if physicians become the final agents in voluntary euthanasia.[19] There is also disagreement about whether euthanasia and assisted suicide should rightly be considered "medical" procedures.[20,21]

Law
Canadian legislation

The Criminal Code of Canada prohibits euthanasia under its homicide provisions, particularly those regarding murder, and makes counselling a person to commit suicide and aiding a suicide punishable offences. The consent of the person whose death is intended docs not alter the criminal nature of these acts.[22]

Canadian case law

In 1993 the Supreme Court of Canada dismissed (by a 5–4 margin) an application by Sue Rodriguez, a 42-year-old woman with amyotrophic lateral sclerosis, for a declaration that the Criminal Code prohibition against aiding or abetting suicide is unconstitutional. Rodriguez claimed that Section 241(b) of the Code violated her rights under the Charter of Rights and Freedoms to liberty and security of the person, to freedom from cruel and unusual treatment and to freedom from discrimination on grounds of disability, since the option of attempting suicide is legally available to nondisabled people.[6] [Editor's note: Recent developments have included the conviction and sentencing of Robert Latimer, the guilty plea of Dr. Maurice Genereux and criminal charges brought against Dr. Nancy Morrison.]

Other jurisdictions

On Sept. 22, 1996, a cancer patient in Australia's Northern Territory became the first person in the world to receive assistance from a physician to commit suicide under specific legislation.[23] [Editor's note: This legislation has since been disallowed.] In The Netherlands, a series of judicial decisions has made euthanasia permissible under certain guidelines since the 1960s, despite the fact that it is still officially a criminal offence. Several legislative initiatives in the US have either been narrowly defeated[24] or have met with a constitutional challenge.[25]

Two federal courts of appeal in the US independently ruled that there is a constitutionally protected right to choose the time and manner of one's death, and that this right includes seeking assistance in committing suicide.[4,5] However, in the summer of 1997 the US Supreme Court overturned these decisions, rejecting the arguments that the right to liberty includes the right to seek the assistance of a physician to commit suicide, and that the laws prohibiting assisted suicide are discriminatory.[26–28] [Editor's note: Therefore, states may pass their own legislation on this matter. At the time of writing, there is legislation permitting euthanasia in Oregon.]

Policy

In 1993, Sawyer and colleagues identified 4 public-policy options available to Canadian physicians with regard to euthanasia and assisted suicide: (a) oppose any change in the legal prohibition; (b) support a modification of the law to permit euthanasia or assisted suicide, or both, under certain circumstances only; (c) support decriminalization on the assumption that there will be legislation to prevent abuse; (d) maintain neutrality.[29] Despite differences of opinion within its membership, the CMA continues to uphold the position that members should not participate in euthanasia and assisted suicide.[30] This policy is consistent with the policies of medical associations throughout the world.[31]

Empirical studies
Perspectives of patients and the public

Requests for euthanasia and assisted suicide do not arise exclusively out of a desire to avoid pain and suffering. Clinical depression,[32] a desire to maintain personal control,[33] fear of being dependent on others[34] and concern about being a burden to loved ones[35] have all been reported as reasons underlying requests for euthanasia and assisted suicide.

In Canada, more than 75% of the general public support voluntary euthanasia and assisted suicide in the case of patients who are unlikely to recover from their illness.[36] But roughly equal numbers oppose these practices for patients with reversible conditions (78% opposed), elderly disabled people who feel they are a burden to others (75% opposed), and elderly people with only minor physical ailments (83% opposed).[37]

Physicians' perspectives and practices

Results of a survey by Kinsella and Verhoef indicate that 24% of Canadian physicians would be willing to practise euthanasia and 23% would be willing to assist in a suicide if these acts were legal.[38] These findings are similar to the results of surveys conducted in the UK[39] and in Australia's Northern Territory.[40] Surveys of physicians in the Australian state of Victoria,[41] as well as recent surveys in Oregon,[42] Washington[31] and Michigan[43] indicated that a majority of physicians in these jurisdictions supported euthanasia and assisted suicide in principle and favoured their decriminalization. Some studies have documented physician participation in euthanasia and assisted suicide.[31,39,44] Physicians in certain specialties (such as palliative care) appear to be less willing to participate in euthanasia and assisted suicide than physicians in other specialties.[25,35,38]

How should I approach euthanasia and assisted suicide in practice?

Euthanasia and assisted suicide violate the Criminal Code of Canada and are punishable by life imprisonment and 14 years in prison, respectively. Physicians who believe that euthanasia and assisted suicide should be legally accepted in Canada should pursue these convictions through the various legal and democratic means at their disposal, i.e., the courts and the legislature. In approaching these issues in a clinical setting it is important to differentiate between: (a) respecting competent decisions to forgo treatment, such as discontinuing mechanical ventilation at the request of a patient who is unable to breathe independently, which physicians may legally do; (b) providing appropriate palliative measures, such as properly titrated pain control, which physicians are obliged to do; and (c) acceding to requests for euthanasia and assisted suicide, both of which are illegal.

The case of Ms. DD involves a competent, terminally ill patient who is imminently dying and in intractable pain. The case of Mr. EE involves an apparently competent patient who is not dying but is experiencing extreme mental suffering.

In both cases the physician is confronted with a request to participate in euthanasia or assisted suicide. The physician should explore the specific reasons behind the request and provide whatever treatment, counselling or comfort measures that may be necessary. For example, for Ms. DD, it may be necessary to seek the advice of a pain specialist about alternative approaches to pain management and palliation. The case of Mr. EE is in many ways more difficult, since depression has been ruled out as a contributing factor in the request. The physician must attempt to investigate and ameliorate any other psychosocial problems that are affecting the patient.

Providing euthanasia and assisted suicide in either case could result in conviction and imprisonment. However, increasing the morphine dosage for Ms. DD as necessary to relieve her pain is lawful, even though it may eventually prove toxic and precipitate death.

References

1. *Of life and death. Report of the Special Senate Committee on Euthanasia and Assisted Suicide.* Ottawa: Supply and Services Canada;1995. p. 14 [cat no YC2-351/1-OIE].
2. Brock DW. Voluntary active euthanasia. *Hastings Cent Rep* 1992;22(2):10-22.
3. *Compassion in dying* v. *Washington*, 79 F 3rd 790 (9th Cir 1996).
4. *Quill* v. *Vacco*, 80 F 3rd 716 (2nd Cir 1996).
5. Rachels J. Active and passive euthanasia. *N Engl J Med* 1975;292:78-80.

6. *Sue Rodriguez* v. *British Columbia (AG)*, [1993] 3 SCR 519. [See Justice Cory's dissent.]

7. Roy DJ. Euthanasia: taking a stand. *J Palliat Care* 1990;6(1):3-5.

8. Dickens BM. Medically assisted death: *Nancy B.* v. *Hôtel-Dieu de Québec*. *McGill Law J* 1993;38:1053-70.

9. Gillon R. Euthanasia, withholding life-prolonging treatment, and moral differences between killing and letting die. *J Med Ethics* 1988;14:115-7.

10. Annas GJ. The promised end: constitutional aspects of physician-assisted suicide. *N Engl J Med* 1996;335:683-7.

11. Quill T. The ambiguity of clinical intentions. *N Engl J Med* 1993;329:1039-40.

12. Brody H. Causing, intending and assisting death. *J Clin Ethics* 1993;4:112-7.

13. Angell M. The Supreme Court and physician-assisted suicide — the ultimate right [editorial]. *N Engl J Med* 1997;336:50-3.

14. Foley KM. Competent care of the dying instead of physician-assisted suicide [editorial]. *N Engl J Med* 1997;336:54-8.

15. Callaghan D. When self-determination runs amok. *Hastings Cent Rep* 1992;22(2):52-5.

16. Brody H. Assisted death: a compassionate response to a medical failure. *N Engl J Med* 1992;327:1384-8.

17. Kamisar Y. Against assisted suicide — even a very limited form. *U Detroit Mercy Law Rev* 1995;72:735-69.

18. Kamisar Y. Some non-religious views against proposed "mercy killing" legislation. *Minnesota Law Rev* 1958;42:969-1042.

19. Quill TE, Cassel CK, Meier DE. Care of the hopelessly ill: proposed clinical criteria for physician-assisted suicide. *N Engl J Med* 1992;327:1380-4.

20. Kinsella DT. Will euthanasia kill medicine? *Ann R Coll Physicians Surg Can* 1991;24(7):489-92.

21. Drickamer MA, Lee MA, Ganzini L. Practical issues in physician-assisted suicide. *Ann Intern Med* 1997;126(2):146-51.

22. *Criminal Code*, RSC 1985, C-46, ss 14, 222, 229, 241.

23. Ryan CJ, Kaye M. Euthanasia in Australia: the Northern Territory Rights of the Terminally Ill Act. *N Engl J Med* 1996;334:326-8.

24. Cohen JS, Fihn SD, Boyko EJ, Jonsen AR, Wood RW. Attitudes toward assisted suicide and euthanasia among physicians in Washington State. *N Engl J Med* 1994;331:89-94.

25. Alpers A, Lo B. Physician-assisted suicide in Oregon. *JAMA* 1995;274:483-7.

26. Lavery JV, Singer PA. The "Supremes" decide on assisted suicide: What should a doctor do? [editorial]. *CMAJ* 1997;154(4):405-6.

27. *Washington* v. *Glucksberg*, 117 S Ct 2302 (1997).

28. *Quill* v. *Vacco*, 117 S Ct 2293 (1997).

29. Sawyer DM, Williams JR, Lowy F. Canadian physicians and euthanasia: 5. Policy options. *CMAJ* 1993;148:2129-33.

30. Canadian Medical Association. Physician-assisted death [policy summary]. *CMAJ* 1995;152:248A-B.

31. Shapiro RS, Derse AR, Gottlieb M, Schiedermayer D, Olson M. Willingness to perform euthanasia: a survey of physician attitudes. *Arch Intern Med* 1994;154:575-84.

32. Chochinov HM, Wilson KG, Enns M, Mowchun N, Lander S, Levitt M, et al. Desire for death in the terminally ill. *Am J Psychiatry* 1995;152:1185-91.

33. Ogden R. *Euthanasia, assisted suicide and AIDS*. Vancouver: Perrault/Goedman Publishing, 1994. p. 58.

34. Back AL, Wallace JI, Starks HE, Pearlman RA. Physician-assisted suicide and

euthanasia in Washington State: patient requests and physician responses. *JAMA* 1996;275:919-25.

35. Emanuel EJ, Fairclough DL, Daniels ER, Clarridge BR. Euthanasia and physician-assisted suicide: attitudes and experiences of oncology patients, oncologists, and the public. *Lancet* 1996;347:1805-10.

36. Singer PA, Choudhry S, Armstrong J, Meslin EM, Lowy F. Public opinion regarding end-of-life decisions: influence of prognosis, practice and process. *Soc Sci Med* 1995;41:1517-21.

37. Genuis SJ, Genuis SK, Chang W. Public attitudes toward the right to die. *CMAJ* 1994;150:701-8.

38. Wysong P. Doctors divided on euthanasia acceptance: preference is to refer euthanasia to another doctor. *Med Post* 1996;32(34):1,90.

39. Ward BJ, Tate PA. Attitudes among NHS doctors to requests for euthanasia. *BMJ* 1994;308:1332-4.

40. Managing a comfortable death [editorial]. *Lancet* 1996;347:1777.

41. Kuhse H, Singer P. Doctors' practices and attitudes regarding voluntary euthanasia. *Med J Aust* 1988;148:623-7.

42. Lee MA, Nelson HD, Tilden VP, Ganzini L, Schmidt TA, Tolle SW. Legalizing assisted suicide — views of physicians in Oregon. *N Engl J Med* 1996;334:310-5.

43. Bachman JG, Alcser KH, Doukas DJ, Lichtenstein RL, Corning AD, Brody H. Attitudes of Michigan physicians and the public toward legalizing physician-assisted suicide and voluntary euthanasia. *N Engl J Med* 1996;334:303-9.

44. Fried TR, Stein MD, O'Sullivan PS, Brock DW, Novack DH. The limits of patient autonomy: physician attitudes and practices regarding life-sustaining treatments and euthanasia. *Arch Intern Med* 1993;153:722-8.

14

Dealing with demands for "inappropriate" treatment: medical futility and other approaches

Charles Weijer, MD, PhD; Peter A. Singer, MD, MPH;
Bernard M. Dickens, PhD, LLD; Stephen Workman, MD, MSc

Mr. FF, a 58-year-old man with metastatic cancer, is admitted to hospital because of sepsis. When his physician discusses a do-not-resuscitate order with him, the patient is adamant that he wants to be resuscitated in the event of cardiac arrest.

Mrs. GG is 43 years old and in a persistent vegetative state secondary to head trauma suffered in a motor vehicle accident 13 months ago. She and her family are Orthodox Jews. When pneumonia develops, the family insists that "everything be done" for her, including, if necessary, treatment in the intensive care unit.

What are demands for inappropriate treatment?

The right of the patient to refuse an unwanted medical intervention, even a life-saving treatment, is a well-established ethical and legal dictum in medicine. The limits of patient autonomy, however, have been challenged recently by demands from patients and families for medical interventions considered by the health care team to be inappropriate. Although treatment demanded by patients runs the gamut of medical interventions, the most pressing cases involve appeals for life-sustaining treatment. Must clinicians always accede to the wishes of patients and families? Are all such cases more or less similar, or are important moral distinctions among cases to be drawn?

A number of approaches to the problem have been proposed. Perhaps the best known is that of "medical futility." The concept was devised to take "precedence over patient autonomy and [permit] physicians to withhold or withdraw care deemed to be inappropriate without subjecting such a decision to patient approval."[1] According to this view, a treatment is quantitatively futile "when physicians conclude (either through personal experience, experiences shared with colleagues, or consideration of reported empiric data) that in the last 100 cases, a medical treatment has been useless." A treatment is qualitatively futile if it "merely preserves permanent unconsciousness or . . . fails to end total dependence on intensive medical care."[1] Futile treatment need neither be offered to patients nor be provided if demanded.

Critics of medical futility have argued that it confounds morally distinct cases: demand for treatment unlikely to work and demand for effective treatment supporting a controversial end (e.g., permanent unconsciousness). They point out that the concept of medical futility is unnecessary in the first case and harmful in the second. Appeals for ineffective treatment can be dismissed because such treatment falls outside the bounds of standard medical care.[2] Cases in which care is effective but the end supported is controversial typically involve substantial value disagreements. An optimal approach to such cases will rest on open communication and negotiation between the health care team and the patient or family.

Why are demands for inappropriate treatment important?

Demands for inappropriate treatment, although infrequent, cause substantial emotional and moral distress for patients, families and health care workers. In a few cases conflict may be so severe that legal action is taken by either the hospital or the patient.

Ethics

Medical care is governed by a number of ethical principles, including respect for persons, beneficence, nonmaleficence and justice.[3] These principles find expression in the CMA's Code of Ethics.[4] When caring for patients, including those who are receiving (or who may receive) life-prolonging treatments, physicians have an obligation to "[a]scertain wherever possible and recognize [the] patient's wishes about the initiation, continuation or cessation of life-sustaining treatment" and, if the patient is unable to speak for himself or herself, to respect wishes expressed in an advance directive or by a proxy decision-maker (usually a family member).[4] Obligations to respect the wishes of patients, however, must be tempered by duties to "consider first the well-being of the patient" and to provide "appropriate care."[4] Finally, physicians must not discriminate against patients on such grounds as medical condition, disability or religion.[4] Demands for ineffective treatment and demands for effective treatment that supports a controversial end must be considered separately.[5]

Demands for ineffective treatment

It is uncontroversial that clinicians have no obligation to provide a treatment that cannot work or is very unlikely to work (e.g., an antibiotic to treat a common cold or mechanical ventilation in the presence of massive tumour deposits in the chest).[5,6] Such treatment falls outside the bounds of "appropriate care." But what of demands for experimental treatment (treatment with an unknown chance of success) when proven treatment exists or treatment is effective but outdated (the success rate is known to be less than that of standard treatment but greater than 1%)? Medical futility provides no basis to refuse these prima facie unreasonable requests from patients. Clearly, then, we require a more robust ethical concept.

"Appropriate care" is most productively understood as treatment that falls within the bounds of standard medical practice, that is, medical interventions used by at least a "respectable minority" of expert practitioners.[7,8] Standard of care is a well-established concept rooted in the physician–patient relationship: "[The] health care professional has an obligation to allow a patient to choose from among medically acceptable treatment options . . . or to reject all options. No one, however, has an obligation to provide interventions that would, in his or her judgement, be countertherapeutic."[9]

Thus, on the basis of standard of care alone, and without appeal to medical futility, clinicians have a sound basis for refusing to provide ineffective, experimental or outdated treatment.

Demands for effective treatment that supports a controversial end

Disagreements about so-called qualitatively futile treatment are not about probabilities — they are about values. Often the question "What sort of life is worth preserving?" is at their core. Although most patients and their families would not choose to prolong life in a profoundly diminished state, some have very good reasons for doing so. For example, members of a variety of religions, including Orthodox Judaism, fundamentalist Protestantism, fundamentalist Islam and conservative Catholicism, believe that the sanctity of human life implies a religious obligation to seek out and obtain life-prolonging medical treatment.[10] The concept of medical futility wrongly tries to "redefine a debate about conflicting values as a debate about medical probabilities. And given that physicians are generally the sole arbiters of medical probability, this amounts to saying to families, 'Your values don't count.'"[11]

A unilateral decision to withhold or withdraw care in such cases violates the obligation to respect the wishes and values of the patient and may constitute discrimination on grounds of physical or mental disability, or religion. Within the constraints of available resources, clinicians must try to deal with such conflicts through open communication and negotiation.

Cases at the boundary

Our analysis implicitly rests on the determination of whether a particular treatment falls within the bounds of standard medical care. A variety of factors may be used to argue for a treatment being considered appropriate: the prevalence of its use by expert clinicians (the threshold being its use by at least a "respectable minority"), licensure by Health Canada's Therapeutic Products Directorate for a specific use, and the existence of high-quality scientific evidence of its safety and efficacy.

The gap between scientific evidence and clinical practice is closing because of initiatives in evidence-based medicine, including clinical practice guidelines. Although the correspondence between evidence and practice is currently less than perfect, high-quality evidence of the effectiveness of a treatment may be sufficient to establish that it falls within the bounds of standard care, assuming adequate resources. A fortiori, clear evidence that a prevalent treatment is positively harmful or ineffective establishes that the treatment is not appropriate medical care.

Law

Although the physician has a legal duty to treat a patient once the physician–patient relationship has been established,[12] this does not imply that the physician must provide *any* treatment demanded by the patient. Picard and Robertson,[13] in their authoritative book *Legal liability of doctors and hospitals in Canada*, concluded that there is no obligation to inform patients of or to provide them with treatment that is completely ineffective.

Nor is there a duty to provide treatment contrary to the patient's best interest. Manitoba's Court of Appeal recently ruled on a case involving a do-not-resuscitate (DNR) order being challenged by the parents of a 1-year-old child in a persistent vegetative state.[14] The child had been savagely attacked at 3 months of age and afterward had been taken by the Child and Family Services of Central Manitoba. Justice J.A. Twaddle, upholding the lower court's decision to grant the DNR order, commented: "[I]t is in no one's interest to artificially maintain the life of a . . . patient who is in an irreversible vegetative state. That is unless those responsible for the patient being in that state have an interest in prolonging life to avoid criminal responsibility for the death."[14] That is, the judge found that the parents were not deciding in the best interest of the child.

A case involving a demand for life-prolonging treatment based on deeply rooted cultural or religious beliefs has yet to be considered by

Canadian courts, and so the issue remains undecided. Defendant doctors and hospitals are likely to be confronted with a number of well-known cases in US courts that have sided with families and supported the provision of life-sustaining treatment, but Canadian courts are not necessarily influenced by these decisions.[15] The US cases of Helga Wanglie and Baby K are particularly well known. Both cases involved demands for continued life-prolonging treatments for patients in a persistent vegetative state. In the Wanglie case, the court refused an attempt to have the husband replaced as the decision-maker for his wife.[16,17] In the Baby K case, the court ordered physicians to provide life-prolonging interventions to the child.[18]

In other US cases courts have sided with clinicians. In the Gilgunn case, a jury found that clinicians were not negligent for the death of a patient when they removed mechanical ventilation despite the objections of the patient's daughter.[19] Commentators have questioned whether the court would have sided against the family if the patient were still alive and the continued provision of life-sustaining care were at issue.[20] The decision by the Court of Appeal of Manitoba is consistent with many others in common-law jurisdictions. In a leading English case, for instance, Lord Keith noted the following: "[A] medical practitioner is under no duty to continue to treat . . . a patient where a large body of informed and responsible medical opinion is to the effect that no benefit would be conferred by continuance."[21]

Policy

Issues raised by demands for inappropriate treatment have been dealt with in a number of policy statements.[22-26] All of these policies acknowledge the patient's right to refuse unwanted medical treatment, even life-prolonging treatment. Some of these policies assert that the physician has a right to unilaterally withhold or withdraw treatment that she or he deems futile. For example, the CMA's "Joint statement on resuscitative interventions (update 1995)" states that "[t]here is no obligation to offer a person futile or nonbeneficial treatment"; that is, the treatment "offers no reasonable hope of recovery or improvement or . . . the person is permanently unable to experience any benefit."[24] The policy was recently criticized on the basis that families of people in a persistent vegetative state may have morally and legally enforceable reasons to demand CPR.[11]

At least one recent policy initiative has shifted away from attempts to define "futility" and has instead focused on the establishment of fair procedures for dealing with demands for inappropriate treatment. This initiative involves a staged approach to such conflicts currently in use in a number of hospitals in Texas.[27] The procedure emphasizes clear communication, negotiation and, if needed, impartial arbitration. The University of Toronto Critical Care Program and Joint Centre for Bioethics have developed a model policy on appropriate use of life-sustaining treatment (www.utoronto.ca/jcb [under "end of life"]).

Empirical studies

Decisions to withhold or withdraw life-sustaining treatment are common in modern health care.[28–30] Disagreements over withdrawing life support, a kind of demand for inappropriate treatment, are relatively uncommon and many resolve over time.[28–30] Demands for inappropriate treatment are nonetheless a source of substantial moral and emotional distress for health care workers and patients' families.[31,32] Such requests and the distress they incite arise from a variety of causes, including unrealistic expectations of the family, failure of the clinician to be realistic, lack of clear explanation of the implications of continued treatment and fear of litigation.[33]

How should I approach demands for inappropriate treatment in practice?

If the proposed treatment clearly falls outside the bounds of standard medical care, the physician has no obligation to offer or provide it. However, if substantial medical controversy as to the beneficial effect of the treatment exists, the law on this issue is unclear. Furthermore, this assertion does not address the emotions surrounding a case, so the clinician should proceed with caution.

Some of the most difficult cases occur at the boundary of appropriate medical care, when it is unclear whether demanded treatment falls within the standard of care. A treatment may have little evidence to support its safety and efficacy, it may be advocated by a very small group of physicians, or new evidence may have arisen questioning established use. Because patients and their families have increased access to uncontrolled sources of medical information on the Internet, demands for treatment of this sort may increase. In such cases, the physician ought to consult with colleagues within and outside of the institution: How prevalent is the treatment? How respected are those advocating it? Is there evidence for efficacy and safety? Beyond these obvious questions, others will need to be asked by the physician: Am I competent to administer the treatment? Does its provision violate my own conscience or the mission of my institution? A negative response to these last 2 questions calls for the patient to be transferred to the care of another physician or another institution.

Misunderstandings, emotional anguish and disagreements about fundamental values often lie at the heart of cases in which seemingly inappropriate care is demanded. Therefore, the health care team should take a patient, supportive, empathic and open approach in attempting to resolve these cases. Effective communication skills are essential. The physician should ask: Why has the conflict over treatment arisen? What are the deeper issues at stake (e.g., a need for more information, denial, trust, differing values)? Such cases often also lead to conflicts among members of the health care team, and these too should be addressed in an open and constructive manner.

When disagreement among health care providers, patient and family persists, the physician should conceptualize this as a situation of conflict in which the goal is to seek a negotiated solution.[34] If necessary, the physician should seek the services of someone trained in conflict mediation, such as a clinical bioethicist, psychiatrist, psychologist or social worker.

If the conflict cannot be resolved through mediation, arbitration may be necessary. Consultation with a lawyer is important at this stage. Some provinces have provisions in their consent laws for arbitration through boards. For example, the Consent and Capacity Board in Ontario has the power to replace a substitute decision-maker who is not making decisions according to the patient's wishes or best interest.[35] As a final recourse, the courts may be appealed to by either party, but this step runs the risk of increasing both the emotional anguish of patients, family and health care providers, and the conflict among them. Ideally, the health care institution will have a policy on dealing with demands for inappropriate treatment. The policy should describe a clear and nonarbitrary process to address such cases in the institution.[27]

Mr. FF has advanced cancer and demands cardiopulmonary resuscitation (CPR). There is good evidence that CPR is very unlikely to be effective for patients with metastatic cancer or sepsis, let alone a patient who has both; therefore, such treatment falls outside the bounds of standard care.[36-39] We have said that, in general, there is no obligation to offer or provide such treatment. Should the decision to withhold CPR be communicated to the patient? We think so. First, the expectation on the part of the patient that CPR will be provided may create an obligation to disclose the fact that it will not be provided and the reasons why.[13] Second, it furthers the end of honest and open communication with the patient. Third, and perhaps most important, it provides the physician with the opportunity to explore the motivations for the demand. If denial is a factor, counselling may be offered. If control is an issue, the clinician should help the patient focus on the various options that exist regarding his care. Clinicians should remain open to the possibility of compassionate exceptions to withholding CPR. For example, if the patient is motivated by the wish to survive to see a relative who will arrive shortly, a time-limited order to attempt resuscitation may be written.

Mrs. GG is in a persistent vegetative state, and her family demands aggressive medical treatment. The disagreement is not about the efficacy of the interventions, but whether they should be used to prolong a state of permanent unconsciousness. Health care workers should not unilaterally refuse to provide treatment in this case. Compromise should be sought through open communication and negotiation. The scarcity of resources, particularly beds in the intensive care unit, is undoubtedly an issue that must be dealt with in this case (and similar cases). An attempt at compromise may include the provision of a variety of treatments outside the intensive care unit, perhaps including fluids, nutrition, physiotherapy, supplemental oxygen and antibiotics.

References

1. Schneiderman LJ, Jecker NS, Jonsen AR. Medical futility: its meaning and ethical implications. *Ann Intern Med* 1990;112:949-54.
2. Weijer C, Elliott C. Pulling the plug on futility. *BMJ* 1995;310:683-4.
3. Beauchamp TL, Childress JF. *Principles of biomedical ethics.* 4th ed. New York: Oxford University Press; 1994.
4. Canadian Medical Association. *Code of ethics.* Ottawa: The Association; 1996.
5. Truog RD, Brett AS, Frader J. The problem with futility. *N Engl J Med* 1992;326:1560-4.
6. *Of life and death. Report of the Special Senate Committee on Euthanasia and Assisted Suicide.* Ottawa: Supply and Services Canada; 1995. Cat no YC2-351/1-OIE.
7. Freedman B, McGill/Boston Research Group. Nonvalidated therapies and HIV disease. *Hastings Cent Rep* 1989;19(3):14-20.
8. Brett AS, McCullough LB. When patients request specific interventions: defining the limits of the physician's obligation. *N Engl J Med* 1986;315:1347-51.
9. US President's Commission for the Study of Ethical Problems in Medicine and Biomedical Research. *Deciding to forgo life-sustaining treatment: a report on the ethical, medical and legal issues in treatment decisions.* Washington: The Commission; 1983.
10. Post SG. Baby K, medical futility and the free exercise of religion. *J Law Med Ethics* 1995;23:20-6.
11. Weijer C. Cardiopulmonary resuscitation for patients in a persistent vegetative state: Futile or acceptable? *CMAJ* 1998;158(4):491-3.
12. Picard EI, Robertson GB. *Legal liability of doctors and hospitals in Canada.* 3rd ed. Scarborough (ON): Carswell; 1996. p. 235-69.
13. Picard EI, Robertson GB. *Legal liability of doctors and hospitals in Canada.* 3rd ed. Scarborough (ON): Carswell; 1996. p. 264-5.
14. *Child and Family Services of Central Manitoba* v. *Lavallee* (14 Nov 1997), (Man CA) [unreported].
15. Daar JF. Medical futility and implications for physician autonomy. *Am J Law Med* 1995;21:221-40.
16. Angell M. The case of Helga Wanglie: a new kind of "right to die" case. *N Engl J Med* 1991;325:511-2.
17. Capron AM. In re Helga Wanglie. *Hastings Cent Rep* 1991;21(5):26-8.
18. Annas GJ. Asking the courts to set the standard of emergency care — the case of Baby K. *N Engl J Med* 1994;330:1542-5.

19. *Gilgunn* v. *Massachusetts General Hospital.* No 92-4820 (Mass Sup Ct Civ Action Suffolk Co 22 Apr 1995).
20. Prip W, Moretti A. Medical futility: a legal perspective. In: Zucker MB, Zucker HD, editors. *Medical futility and the evaluation of life-sustaining interventions.* Cambridge (MA): Cambridge University Press; 1997. p. 136-54.
21. *Airedale N.H.S. Trust* v. *Bland* [1993] 1 All ER 821 at 861.
22. American Thoracic Society Bioethics Task Force. Withholding and withdrawing life-sustaining therapy. *Am Rev Respir Dis* 1991;144:726-31.
23. Society of Critical Care Medicine Ethics Committee. Consensus statement on the triage of critically ill patients. *JAMA* 1994;271:1200-3.
24. Joint statement on resuscitative interventions (update 1995). *CMAJ* 1995;153(11):1652A-C.
25. Murphy DJ, Barbour E. GUIDe (Guidelines for the Use of Intensive care in Denver): a community effort to define futile and inappropriate care. *New Horiz* 1994;2:326-30.
26. Task Force on Ethics of the Society of Critical Care Medicine. Consensus on the ethics of forgoing life-sustaining treatments in the critically ill. *Crit Care Med* 1990;18:1435-9.
27. Halevy A, Brody BA. A multi-institution collaborative policy on medical futility. *JAMA* 1996;276:571-4.
28. Wood GG, Martin E. Withholding and withdrawing life-sustaining therapy in a Canadian intensive care unit. *Can J Anaesth* 1995;42:186-91.
29. Prendergast TJ, Luce JM. Increasing incidence of withholding and withdrawal of life support from the critically ill. *Am J Respir Crit Care Med* 1997;155:15-20.
30. Corley MC. Moral distress of critical care nurses. *Am J Crit Care* 1995;4:280-5.
31. Solomon MZ. How physicians talk about futility: making words mean too many things. *J Clin Ethics* 1993;21:231-7.
32. Simmonds A. Decision-making by default: experiences of physicians and nurses with dying patients in intensive care. *Humane Health Care Int* 1996;12:168-72.
33. McCrary SV, Swanson JW, Younger SJ, Perkins HS, Winslade WJ. Physicians' quantitative assessments of medical futility. *J Clin Ethics* 1994;5:100-5.
34. Fisher R, Ury W. *Getting to yes: negotiating agreement without giving in.* New York: Penguin; 1991.
35. *Health Care Consent Act,* SO 1996, c 2, sch A.
36. Bedell SE, Delbanco TL, Cook EF, Epstein FH. Survival after cardiopulmonary resuscitation in the hospital. *N Engl J Med* 1983;309:569-76.
37. Warner SC, Sharma TK. Outcome of cardiopulmonary resuscitation and predictors of resuscitation status in an urban community teaching hospital. *Resuscitation* 1994;27:13-21.
38. Ballew KA, Philbrick JT, Caven DE, Schorling JB. Predictors of survival following in-hospital cardiopulmonary resuscitation. A moving target. *Arch Intern Med* 1994;154:2426-32.
39. Schultz SC, Cullinane DC, Pasquale MD, Magnant C, Evans SR. Predicting in-hospital mortality during cardiopulmonary resuscitation. *Resuscitation* 1996;33:13-7.

Authors' note: Dr. Weijer's research is supported by an Operating Grant and Scholar Award from the Medical Research Council of Canada.

15

Quality end-of-life care

Peter A. Singer, MD, MPH; Neil MacDonald, CM, MD

A physician is sitting at home enjoying dinner when the phone rings. The caller is Mr. HH, an acquaintance. He is distraught. He asks how much air must be injected into an intravenous line to cause a person to die. When asked why he wants to know, he explains that his 72-year-old father, currently a patient in a local hospital, has end-stage metastatic lung cancer and is in excruciating pain. Mr. HH cannot bear to see his father in such pain and wants to end his suffering by means of an air embolism.

Mr. II, a 68-year-old man with a 100 pack-year history of smoking and known chronic obstructive pulmonary disease, presents to the emergency department with pneumonia and respiratory failure. He has been intubated 4 times before for respiratory failure. He uses oxygen at home and is dyspneic at rest. He has hypoxemia and hypercapnia and is delirious. The emergency physician tries to stabilize his condition with oxygen, salbutamol, steroids and noninvasive ventilation, but Mr. II's respiratory status worsens. Unable to locate the patient's family, the emergency physician calls his family physician and respirologist to find out whether they have ever discussed reintubation, but unfortunately neither has done so. Although she is uncomfortable with this situation because of the uncertainty about the patient's wishes, the emergency physician decides to perform the intubation.

What is end-of-life care?

A physician who receives a call from the emergency department to see a patient with heart failure will have a clear concept of what heart failure is, as well as a framework within which to approach the condition and its management. Our thesis is that physicians do not have an analogous conceptual framework for approaching end-of-life care. Several aspects of end-of-life care are addressed in other chapters, especially those on truth telling (chapter 7), consent (chapter 1), capacity (chapter 3), substitute decision-making (chapter 5), advance care planning (chapter 6), euthanasia and assisted suicide (chapter 13) and appropriate use of life-sustaining treatment (chapter 14). Our purpose here is to incorporate these pieces into a coherent conceptual framework that physicians can use to approach the care of patients at the end of life. Our framework, described in greater detail in the section "How should I approach end-of-life care in practice?," has 3 main elements: control of pain and other symptoms, decisions on the use of life-sustaining treatment, and support of dying patients and their families. This chapter underlines the primary purpose of this book as outlined in the Preface: "to elucidate key concepts in bioethics and to help clinicians to integrate bioethical knowledge into daily practice. . . . [T]he goal is to support performance: what clinicians actually do".

Why is end-of-life care important?

Ethics and law

From an ethical perspective, the principle of beneficence requires that pain and other symptoms be controlled. The legal status of control of pain and other symptoms is not absolutely clear, but physicians should not risk legal peril if they follow established guidelines distinguishing these practices from euthanasia.[1]

Aspects of "life-sustaining treatment" comprise advance care planning, decisions to withhold or withdraw life-sustaining treatment and appropriate use of life-sustaining treatment. Advance care planning is ethically supported by the principle of respect for autonomy and is legally recognized in most Canadian provinces (see chapter 6). Decisions by patients or substitute decision-makers to withhold or withdraw life-sustaining treatment proposed by a physician are supported by the ethical principle of respect for autonomy and the legal doctrine of informed consent (see chapters 1, 3 and 5). In contrast, the ethical and legal issues related to appropriate use of life-sustaining treatments demanded by patients and substitute decisions-makers over the objections of physicians are not as clear (see chapter 14). Both euthanasia and assisted suicide are illegal in Canada (see chapter 13).

Policy

Recent policy initiatives have framed end-of-life care as an issue in health care quality — a positive development, in that it focuses organizational commitment to quality on the problem of end-of-life care. But what does quality end-of-life care entail? In the United States, several organizations have published a "statement of principles" of quality end-of-life care that includes the following domains: treatment of physical and emotional symptoms, support of function and autonomy, advance care planning, aggressive care near death, patient and family satisfaction, global quality of life, family burden, survival time, provider continuity and skill, and bereavement.[2] The Committee on Care at the End of Life of the US Institute of Medicine, National Academy of Sciences, has proposed the following 6 categories of quality end-of-life care: overall quality of life, physical well-being and functioning, psychosocial well-being and functioning, spiritual well-being, patient perception of care, and family well-being and perceptions.[3]

Empirical studies

Although euthanasia consumes the attention of the media, the critical ethical issues vexing physicians, patients and families lie elsewhere. In particular, pain is often poorly managed.[4-6] In a study of older patients who were conscious during the last 3 days of life, 4 in 10 had severe pain most of the time.[7] In a survey of physicians and nurses at 5 US hospitals, 47% of respondents reported that they had acted against their conscience in providing care to the terminally ill, and 55% reported that they sometimes felt the treatments they offered patients were overly burdensome.[8]

Consistent with the recent focus of policy efforts, quality improvement strategies have been applied at the organizational level to the problem of end-of-life care.[9,10] For example, in an innovative program called "Dialogue to Action," Jacobson and associates[11] arranged for the next of kin of patients who had died to describe their experiences of end-of-life care to members of the hospital ethics committee. It is likely that appropriate organizational change will require both the elicitation of "actionable reports" — narratives of care that highlight specific clinical areas for improvement — as well as the development of innovative ways to change clinical practice, for instance, by focusing traditional "morbidity and mortality rounds" on quality end-of-life care.

How should I approach end-of-life care in practice?

To address this question, we recommend a conceptual framework with 3 main elements: control of pain and other symptoms, decisions on the use of life-sustaining treatments, and support of dying patients and their families. We do not believe that a conceptual framework will magically solve the documented problems in end-of-life care; we do, however, believe that this is an important step.

Control of pain and other symptoms

No patient should die in pain or with other treatable symptoms. Indeed, before social, psychosocial and spiritual problems can be properly addressed, good symptom control must first be achieved: it is difficult to contemplate spiritual issues or to reflect on life's accomplishments when in pain or with kidney basin in hand. The undertreatment of pain and other symptoms is well documented, but aside from inadequate training of health professionals[12,13] the causes are complicated and not well understood. On occasion, physicians may be concerned about balancing good symptom control with the risk of hastening death. Guidelines have been developed to assist physicians in distinguishing appropriate analgesia from euthanasia by lethal injection.[1] Controlling other symptoms, such as nausea, fatigue and breathlessness, may be even more challenging than controlling pain, but effective approaches have been developed.[14]

Physicians must keep in mind that the problems of dying patients have their genesis at an earlier time in the trajectory of illness. Thus, palliative care should not be isolated as simply an end-of-life option; it must be intermeshed with therapies aimed at prolongation of life or cure. As in other areas of medicine, prevention or early control of a symptom is preferable to a rescue attempt on preventable, but now out-of-control, suffering. Every physician who cares for dying patients should ensure that he or she has adequate skills in this domain, as well as access to skilled consultative help from palliative care specialists. A list of leading journals and other information sources is given at the end of this chapter.

Use of life-sustaining treatments

To the extent possible, the patient and his or her family should be able to choose the setting and nature of the care that the patient will receive in the last days of life and should be encouraged to discuss in advance their desires regarding life-sustaining treatments and personal care. Physicians should facilitate this advance care planning (see chapter 6)[15–18] and guide and support the patient and the family through the process of giving consent to treatment and arranging for substitute decision-making (see chapter 5). A key skill here is the communication of bad news.[19] In addition, physicians need to develop an approach to the opposite problem — when the patient or the family demands treatment that the physician feels is inappropriate (see chapter 14). The key here is the ability to negotiate a treatment plan that is acceptable to the patient, the family and the health care team.[20]

Support of patients and their families

The support that each patient and his or her family needs from the physician is unique. The best way to find out what support will be appropriate in a particular situation is to ask, "How can I help you?"

Attention to psychosocial issues demands involvement of the patients and their families as partners. Although physicians should be sensitive to the range of psychosocial distress and social disruption common to dying patients and their families, they may not be as available or as skilled as nurses, social workers and other health care professionals in addressing certain issues. An interdisciplinary health care team can help in these areas.

Spiritual issues often come to the fore as one is dying, and pastoral care teams should be available to assist the patient's own clergy in counselling.

Although not all families need or desire follow-up after the death of a loved one, many appreciate a letter or a telephone call from the physician or a member of the palliative care team. Some families will need more specific help. Physicians should be sensitive to risk factors for poor adjustment to bereavement and should be knowledgeable about local bereavement services.[21]

Both of the cases we have presented represent failures in end-of-life care. In the first, inadequate pain control led to a desire for euthanasia. What was needed was not an air embolism but better pain control. When this was achieved, Mr. HH was relieved and did not pursue the idea of euthanasia. This case also illustrates that physicians should not take requests for euthanasia at face value; rather, they should explore and address the problems in end-of-life care that might have led to such requests.

The second case represents a failure of communication about life-sustaining treatments. Mr. II had end-stage lung disease and had been intubated 4 times previously, so he was ideally situated to know whether he wanted to undergo the procedure again; indeed, it is very likely that he had considered this possibility. If he did want intubation, knowledge of his wishes would have relieved the emergency physician's anxiety. (Although death was looming, it would be difficult to claim that intubation would be futile in this case, given that it had worked before.) If Mr. II did not want to undergo intubation, he missed his opportunity to communicate this desire. Arguably, the family physician and the respirologist should have broached this issue with him and helped him to make his wishes known in such a way that they would be effectively communicated when respiratory failure occurred.

In summary, physicians caring for patients at the end of their lives should ask themselves 3 questions: Am I managing this patient's pain and other symptoms adequately? Have I addressed the relevant issues with respect to the use of life-sustaining treatment? Am I supporting this person and his or her family?

References

1. Lavery JV, Singer PA. The "Supremes" decide on assisted suicide: What should a doctor do? *CMAJ* 1997;157(4):405-6.
2. Measuring quality of care at the end of life: a statement of principles. *J Am Geriatr Soc* 1997;45:526-7.

3. Committee on Care at the End of Life, Institute of Medicine, National Academy of Sciences (Field MJ, Cassel CK, editors). *Approaching death: improving care at the end of life*. Washington: National Academy Press; 1997. p. 142.

4. Cleeland CS, Gonin R, Hatfield AK, Edmonson JH, Blum RH, Stewart JA, et al. Pain and its treatment in outpatients with metastatic cancer. *N Engl J Med* 1994;330:592-6.

5. Portenoy RK, Miransky J, Thaler HT, Hornung J, Bianchi C, Cibas-Kong I, et al. Pain in ambulatory patients with lung or colon cancer. *Cancer* 1992;70:1616-24.

6. Writing Group for SUPPORT Investigators. A controlled trial to improve care for seriously ill hospitalized patients: the Study to Understand Prognoses and Preferences for Outcomes and Risks of Treatments (SUPPORT). *JAMA* 1995;274:1591-8.

7. Lynn J, Teno JM, Phillips RS, Wu AW, Desbiens N, Harrold J, et al. Perceptions by family members of the dying experience of older and seriously ill patients. *Ann Intern Med* 1997;126:97-106.

8. Solomon MZ, O'Donnell L, Jennings B, Guilfoy V, Wolf SM, Nolan K, et al. Decisions near the end of life: professional views on life-sustaining treatments. *Am J Public Health* 1993;83:14-23.

9. Cleary PD, Edgman-Levitan S. Health care quality: incorporating consumer perspectives. *JAMA* 1997;278:1608-12.

10. Baker GR. Collaborating for improvement: the Institute for Healthcare Improvement's breakthrough series. *New Med* 1997;1:5-8.

11. Jacobson JA, Francis LP, Battin MP, Green DJ, Grammes C, VanRiper J, et al. Dialogue to action: lessons learned from some family members of deceased patients at an interactive program in seven Utah hospitals. *J Clin Ethics* 1997;8:359-71.

12. MacDonald N, Findlay HP, Bruera E, Dudgeon D, Kramer J. A Canadian survey of issues in cancer pain management. *J Pain Symptom Manage* 1997;14:332-42.

13. Van Roenn JH, Cleeland CS, Gonin R, Hatfield AK, Pandya KJ. Physician attitudes and practice in cancer pain management. *Ann Intern Med* 1993;119:121-6.

14. Bruera E, Neumann CM. Management of specific symptom complexes in patients receiving palliative care. *CMAJ* 1998;158(13):1717-26.

15. Teno JM, Nelson HL, Lynn J. Advance care planning: priorities for ethical and empirical research. *Hastings Cent Rep* 1994;24(6):S32-6.

16. Emanuel LL, Danis M, Pearlman RA, Singer PA. Advance care planning as a process: structuring the discussions in practice. *J Am Geriatr Soc* 1995;43:440-6.

17. Singer PA, Martin DK, Lavery JV, Thiel EC, Kelner M, Mendelssohn DC. Reconceptualizing advance care planning from the patient's perspective. *Arch Intern Med* 1998;158:879-84.

18. Martin DK, Thiel EC, Singer PA. A new model of advance care planning: observations from people with HIV. *Arch Intern Med*. In press.

19. Buckman R. *How to break bad news: a guide for health care professionals*. Downsview (ON): University of Toronto Press; 1992.

20. Fisher R, Ury W. *Getting to yes: negotiating agreement without giving in*. 2nd ed. New York: Penguin Books; 1991.

21. Parkes CM. Bereavement. In: Doyle D, Hanks GWC, MacDonald N, editors. *Oxford textbook of palliative medicine*. 2nd ed. New York: Oxford University Press; 1998. p. 995-1010.

Resources for physicians providing end-of-life care

Comprehensive textbook

Doyle D, Hanks GWC, MacDonald N, editors. *Oxford textbook of palliative medicine*. 2nd ed. New York: Oxford University Press; 1998.

Palliative care manuals

MacDonald N, Boisvert M, Dudgeon D, Hagen N, editors. *Palliative medicine: a case-based manual.* Oxford: Oxford University Press; 1998.

Regnard C, Hockley J. *Flow diagrams in advanced cancer and other diseases.* London: Edward Arnold; 1995.

Twycross RG. *Symptom management in advanced cancer.* New York and Oxford: Radcliffe Medical Press; 1997.

Weller A, Caroline NL. *Handbook of palliative care in cancer.* Toronto: Butterworth-Heinemann; 1996.

Woodruff R. *Palliative medicine: symptomatic and supportive care for patients with advanced cancer and AIDS.* 2nd ed. Melbourne: Asperula; 1996.

Palliative care standards and policy statements

Canadian Palliative Care Association Standards Committee (Ferris FD, Cummings I, editors). *Palliative care: towards a consensus in standardized principles of practice* [first-phase working document]. Ottawa: Canadian Palliative Care Association; 1995.

Committee on Care at the End of Life, Division of Health Care Services, Institute of Medicine (Field MJ, Cassel CK, editors). *Approaching death: improving care at the end of life.* Washington: National Academy Press; 1997.

Journals

European Journal of Palliative Care
Journal of Pain and Symptom Management
Journal of Palliative Care
Pain
Palliative Medicine
Psycho-Oncology (journal of the psychological, social and behavioural dimensions of cancer)
Supportive Care in Cancer (official journal of the Multinational Association of Supportive Care in Cancer)

Web sites

American Medical Association Education for Physicians on End-of-Life Care: www.ama-assn.org/EPEC

Association québécoise des soins palliatifs: www.aqsp.org/

DeathNET: www.islandnet.com/deathnet

Edmonton Palliative Care Group: www.palliative.org

George Washington University Center to Improve Care of the Dying: www.gwu.edu/~cicd

Oncopain, a forum on pain management open to health care professionals only: www.multi-med.com/oncology/oncopain

Open Society Institute Project on Death in America: www.soros.org/death.html

Robert Wood Johnson Foundation Last Acts Campaign: lastacts.rwjf.org/default_home.htm
University of Ottawa Institute of Palliative Care: www.pallcare.org
University of Toronto Joint Centre for Bioethics (includes the full-text version of the
    Centre's *Living Will* and links to other end-of-life Web sites): www.utoronto.ca/jcb

16

Resource allocation

Martin F. McKneally, MD, PhD; Bernard M. Dickens, PhD, LLD;
Eric M. Meslin, PhD; Peter A. Singer, MD, MPH

Mr. JJ is a 21-year-old computer programmer with cystic fibrosis. Chronic rejection and poorly controlled fungal infections are destroying the lungs he received 15 months ago. He has intermittently required positive-pressure ventilation to maintain adequate oxygenation during flare-ups of infection or rejection. Mr. JJ has been listed as a candidate for a second transplant. However, given the presence of infection and the risks associated with repeat transplantation, his predicted chance of survival is 65% at 1 month and 38% at 24 months.[1]

Mrs. KK is a 42-year-old schoolteacher. She has been listed as a candidate for double lung transplantation because of rapidly progressing pulmonary hypertension associated with hemoptysis and hypoxemia. She is unable to manage at home because of decompensated right heart failure unresponsive to maximal therapy. As a first-time lung transplant candidate who is free of infection, Mrs. KK has a predicted chance of survival of 82% at 1 month and 62% at 2 years.[1]

The surgeon has 1 matching donor organ available for these 2 patients. He knows that the best outcome can be achieved by transplanting both lungs of the donor into the same patient.[2]

When 63-year-old Mr. LL is brought to the emergency department with severe but potentially reversible brain injury after a motor vehicle accident, the attending physician considers going through the charts of each patient in the intensive care unit (ICU) in the hope of finding someone whose need for intensive care is less than that of Mr. LL. She also considers sending Mr. LL to the floor, but knows that this will overtax the capabilities of the floor staff, who are not prepared to manage the patient's elevated intracranial pressure and seizures. Because of recent hospital closures in the region, no other facility is available to share responsibility for the care of patients with neurosurgical problems of this magnitude.

⌐ What is resource allocation?

Resource allocation is the distribution of goods and services to programs and people. In the context of health care, macroallocations of resources are made by governments at the national, provincial and municipal levels. Meso-allocations are made at the level of institutions; for example, hospitals allocate their resources to programs such as cancer treatment, cardiology and dialysis. Microallocations are made at the level of the individual patient. Although these 3 levels are interrelated, in this chapter we focus on resource allocation from the perspective of the practising physician.

Commodity scarcity, illustrated by the lung-transplant cases, is a shortage of a finite resource (such as an organ) because of natural limits to the availability of that resource. Fiscal scarcity, illustrated by the intensive care case, is a shortage of funds.[3]

Why is resource allocation important?

Rising public and professional expectations, an expanding pool of treatable patients and costly new technology must be balanced against tightly monitored health care budgets, competing government priorities and provincial deficits. Ethics, law, policy and empirical studies provide insights that can help clinicians as they try to distribute health care resources fairly.

Ethics

The ethics of resource allocation may be considered in relation to the concept of justice and the physician's fiduciary duty toward the patient.

According to Aristotle's principle of distributive justice, equals should be treated equally and those who are unequal should be treated unequally. Unequal treatment is justified when resources are allocated in light of morally relevant differences, such as those pertaining to need or likely benefit.[4] Characteristics such as sex, sexual orientation, religion, level of education or age alone are morally irrelevant criteria for resource allocation. Because there is no overarching theory of justice to balance competing claims between morally relevant criteria such as need and benefit, fair, open and publicly defensible resource allocation procedures are critical.

The lack of a comprehensive theory of justice gives rise to unresolved issues in rationing; these have been categorized by Daniels[5] as follows.

- The fair chances versus best outcomes problem. To what degree should producing the best outcome be favoured over giving every patient an opportunity to compete for limited resources?
- The priorities problem. How much priority should we give to treating the sickest or most disabled patients?

- The aggregation problem. When should we allow an aggregation of modest benefits to larger numbers of people to outweigh more significant benefits to fewer people?
- The democracy problem. When must we rely on a fair democratic process as the only way to determine what constitutes a fair rationing outcome?[5]

These questions help to frame discussions of resource allocation issues and the development of policies and practices that balance the obligations of physicians as citizens in a just society with their obligations to individual patients.

The power imbalance that exists between physician and patient creates a fiduciary duty on the physician's part to promote the patient's best interest. The extent of this ethical duty, which is fundamental to the physician's role in resource allocation, is a matter of controversy. For instance, Levinsky has argued that "physicians are required to do everything that they believe may benefit each patient without regard to costs or other societal considerations."[6] By contrast, Morreim has argued that "the physician's obligations to the patient can no longer be a single-minded, unequivocal commitment but rather must reflect a balancing. Patients' interests must be weighed against the legitimate competing claims of other patients, of payers, of society as a whole, and sometimes even of the physician himself."[7]

Law

The Canadian Charter of Rights and Freedoms prohibits discrimination on various grounds, including physical or mental disability. It applies only to governmental agencies, not to physicians or to hospitals' internal management decisions.[8] When hospitals implement governmental policies or discharge governmental duties under authority of legislation, however, the government must ensure that its Charter obligations are met.[9]

The federal Charter of Rights and Freedoms and human rights codes in several provinces prohibit discrimination on the basis of race, ethnicity, place of origin, religion, age, sex, sexual orientation and physical or mental disability. Evidence that resources were allocated purely on such grounds could lead to an inquiry and legal proceedings by a court or provincial human rights commission. However, it is not clear how a court or commission could challenge a physician's clinical assessment of a patient's eligibility for a particular treatment. Evidence might be needed of a systematic policy of discrimination or bias against a particular group on the part of the practitioner or institution[10] or government.

In the Eldridge case, for instance, the Supreme Court of Canada held that governmental refusal to spend 0.0025% of the provincial health care budget (i.e., $150 000) to provide sign language interpretation was unlawful discrimination. The Court found that the deaf patients' claim was "not for a benefit that the government, in the exercise of its discretion to allocate resources to address various social problems, has chosen not to provide. On the contrary, they asked only for equal access to services that are available to all."[11]

Courts have been extremely reluctant to become involved in how physicians, hospital and health authorities use their resources. As a British judge has observed, "Difficult and agonizing judgments have to be made as to how a limited budget is best allocated to the maximum advantage of the maximum number of patients. That is not a judgment which the court can make."[12]

Nevertheless, the trial judge in a case heard in British Columbia criticized physicians for offering the explanation that they felt too constrained by the provincial medical insurance plan and their provincial medical association's standards to order a diagnostic CT scan. Although a finding of negligence was made on other grounds, the judge noted that whereas physicians may consider the financial impact of their decisions, financial considerations cannot be decisive. The physician's first duty is to the patient.[13]

It is understood in law that although there is no liability for making a decision that proves to be wrong,[14] there may be liability for making a decision *wrongly*. A decision is made wrongly if demands for economy distort the physician's judgement with respect to the care that is owed to the patient. An error in clinical judgement is not actionable, because the risk of being wrong is inherent in every exercise of judgement. However, to take decisive account of secondary concerns and subordinate the primary concern of care — the patient's well-being — to a budgetary issue is the wrong way for a physician to make a treatment decision. In contrast, governments have the power, and responsibility, to consider financial aspects of overall resource allocation.

Policy

Governments cannot evade their responsibilities under the Charter of Rights and Freedoms by implementing policy through private doctors or public hospitals. Accordingly, physicians must give effect to directives governments issue in discharge of Charter duties, namely of nondiscrimination. Hospitals are not entirely free to spend their global budget as they wish. Clear, fair and widely accepted institutional or professional policies can provide guidance for physicians who are faced with difficult resource allocation decisions. Policies developed for the allocation of organs have reduced conflict between teams and helped prioritize recipients within organ transplantation programs, using generally accepted and publicly reviewed principles and guidelines.[15]

In Oregon, a priority list of treatments is being developed by citizens' committees with input from physicians. This evolving experiment in public policy ranks health care services on the basis of effectiveness and perceived value to the community. Public funds are assigned by the government to make services "above the funding line" available to citizens "below the poverty line."[16] Public funds assigned by the government to pay for health care are spent on treatments according to their priority on the list. Through multiple iterations and public debate, this experiment is producing a useful model for engaging stakeholders from government, the medical profession and the public in the process of health policy development.[17,18]

In Canada, the CMA has provided a framework for decision-making on core and comprehensive health care services that incorporates 3 major dimensions: quality, economics and ethics.[19] As well, Deber and colleagues have proposed a "four-screen" model based on effectiveness, appropriateness, informed choice and public provision.[20] Finally, the CMA' s Code of Ethics states that physicians should "recognize [their] responsibility to promote fair access to health care resources" and should "use health care resources prudently."[21]

Empirical studies

Given the importance of resource allocation decisions in health care today, there is a surprising lack of empirical studies on this topic. In contrast to the hundreds of published studies on advance directives,[22] for example, fewer than 2 dozen empirical studies on resource allocation (excluding cost-effectiveness analyses of various diagnostic tests and treatments) came to light in our literature search. In this section we review some of these studies with reference to the primary question they address.

Is resource allocation occurring now? In a study of dialysis referrals, Mendelssohn and colleagues found that 67% of Ontario physicians believed rationing of dialysis was occurring at the time of the survey and 91% believed that such rationing would occur in the future.[23]

How do health care providers make resource allocation decisions? This question has been addressed by survey methods in the context of dialysis,[23] transplantation,[24-26] rural medicine,[27] and critical care.[28] For instance, a survey by the Society of Critical Care Medicine found that critical care physicians considered quality of life as viewed by the patient, probability of survival, the reversibility of the acute disorder and the nature of any chronic disorder as important factors in deciding which patients to admit to the intensive care unit.[28]

Do people consider age a relevant variable in health care resource allocation? In a survey of public opinion in the United States, Zweibel and colleagues[29] found that most people accept the withholding of life-prolonging medical care from some critically ill older patients, but few would categorically withhold such care on the basis of age alone.

How do decision-makers balance concerns of efficiency and equity? Ubel and collaborators[30] surveyed prospective jurors, medical ethicists and experts in medical decision-making to explore the trade-off between cost-effectiveness and equity in the setting of budget constraints. Many respondents said they would choose a less cost-effective test for the entire population over a more cost-effective test for half the population. Similarly, in a survey of public opinion in Australia, Nord and associates[31] found that a policy of maximizing cost-effectiveness received very limited support when the consequence was a loss of equity and access to services for elderly people and for people with limited potential for improving their health. In other words, equity was valued above cost-effectiveness in both of these surveys.

How should I approach resource allocation in practice?

The clinician's goal is to provide optimal care within the limits imposed by the allocation of resources to health care generally and to the institution, program and specific situation in which an individual patient is treated. The acceptance of such limits is a source of controversy and strong feelings. Baltzan has argued that recognizing limits is a violation of the fiduciary duty to put the individual patient's interest first.[32] Levinsky has eloquently advocated the view that physicians have a duty to "do everything that may benefit each patient without regard to costs or other societal consideration."[6] These are generous and noble, but unrealistic, proposals; the decision to limit the extent of expenditures for some patients in some circumstances is inescapable if we are to justly allocate the resources of the community for the overall good of its members. Morreim aptly compares it to a decision to "abide by the law of gravity."[7] She proposes a clarifying distinction that can ease the moral discomfort of conscientious physicians faced with rationing decisions. She argues persuasively that physicians can generously dispense what is theirs to control and to give — their knowledge, care, skill and diligence — but they must turn to society for dispensation of technologic and other costly resources.[7] Physicians are not a special class of citizens who have the right to allocate resources they do not own and are beyond their control.

The following guidelines may prove helpful in practice.

- Choose interventions known to be beneficial on the basis of evidence of effectiveness.
- Minimize the use of marginally beneficial tests or marginally beneficial interventions.
- Seek the tests or treatments that will accomplish the diagnostic or therapeutic goal for the least cost.
- Advocate for one's own patients but avoid manipulating the system to gain unfair advantage to them.

- Resolve conflicting claims for scarce resources justly, on the basis of morally relevant criteria such as need (e.g., the patient's risk of death or serious harm could be reduced by the treatment) and benefit (e.g., published evidence of effectiveness), using fair and publicly defensible procedures (ideally, incorporating public input).
- Inform patients of the impact of cost constraints on care, but do so in a sensitive way. Blaming administrative or governmental systems during discussions with the patient at the point of treatment should be avoided; it undermines care by reducing confidence and increasing anxiety at a time when the patient is most vulnerable.
- Seek resolution of unacceptable shortages at the level of hospital management (mesoallocation) or government (macroallocation).
- Be prepared to bring patients' complaints of discrimination for denied services to the attention of governmental authorities.

Mrs. KK should receive the double lung transplant. Although her need is approximately equal to that of Mr. JJ, her ability to benefit is substantially greater. The surgeon knows from sound empirical evidence that repeat lung transplantation has a poor prognosis, particularly when chronic infection exists.[1] He can minimize recriminations related to the team members' feelings of loyalty toward Mr. JJ if the transplantation program policy clearly spells out specific and fair procedures to follow when difficult allocation decisions must be made involving similarly deserving patients.

The attending physician should provide reassurance and appropriate care for Mr. LL in the emergency department, as this is the only facility available. If she chooses to discuss the role of cost constraints with the patient or his family, she should do so in a sensitive way that does not undermine their confidence that he will receive the care he needs. She should involve the administrator on call to bring in additional skilled personnel to provide interim care in the emergency department and to help her arrange for the patient's transfer to a facility prepared to care for him. In this way, she clarifies the responsibility of the hospital as a community institution to resolve the mesoallocation problem at an administrative level. The hospital may in turn address the macroallocation of resources at the provincial or regional level through its representatives to the government. The physician should not attempt to resolve problems of this magnitude on her own and should not compromise the care of Mr. LL. She may choose to contribute to the resolution of similar problems in the longer term by making suggestions about system reform to the health ministry or helping with appeals for public support of additional facilities.

References

1. Novick RJ, Kaye MP, Patterson GA, Andréassian B, Klepetko W, Menkis AH, et al. Redo lung transplantation: a North American–European experience. *J Heart Lung Transplant* 1993;12:5-16.

2. DeHoyos AL, Patterson GA, Maurer JR, Ramirez JC, Miller JD, Winton TL. Pulmonary transplantation: early and late results of the Toronto Lung Transplant Group. *J Thorac Cardiovasc Surg* 1992;103:295-306.

3. Morreim EH. *Balancing act: the new medical ethics of medicine's new economics.* Washington: Georgetown University Press; 1995. p. 47-51.

4. Doyal L. Needs, rights, and the moral duties of clinicians. In: Gillon R, Lloyd A, editors. *Principles of health care ethics.* Chichester (NY): John Wiley & Sons; 1994. p. 217-30.

5. Daniels N. Four unsolved rationing problems: a challenge. *Hastings Cent Rep* 1994;24(4):27-9.

6. Levinsky NG. The doctor's master. *N Engl J Med* 1984;311:1573-5.

7. Morreim EH. *Balancing act: the new medical ethics of medicine's new economics.* Washington: Georgetown University Press; 1995. p. 2.

8. *Stoffman* v. *Vancouver General Hospital* (1990), 76 DLR (4th) 700 (SCC).

9. *Eldridge* v. *British Columbia (AG)* (1997), 151 DLR (4th) 577 (SCC).

10. *Korn* v. *Potter* (1996), 134 DLR (4th) 437 (BCSC).

11. *Eldridge* v. *British Columbia (AG)* (1997), 151 DLR (4th) 577 at 630 (SCC).

12. *R.* v. *Cambridge Health Authority,* [1995] 2 All ER 129 at 137 (CA).

13. *Law Estate* v. *Simice* (1994), 21 CCLT (2d) 228 (BCSC).

14. *Whitehouse* v. *Jordan,* [1981] 1 All ER 267 (HL).

15. Hauptman PJ, O'Connor KJ. Medical progress procurement and allocation of solid organs for transplantation. *N Engl J Med* 1997;336:422-31.

16. Hadorn DC. Setting health care priorities in Oregon: cost-effectiveness meets the rule of rescue. *JAMA* 1991;265:2218-25.

17. Garland MJ. Oregon's contribution to defining adequate health care. In: Chapman AR, editor. *Health care reform: a human rights approach.* Washington: Georgetown University Press; 1994. p. 211-32.

18. Kitzhaber J, Kemmy AM. On the Oregon trail [review]. *Br Med Bull* 1995;51:808-18.

19. Canadian Medical Association. *Core and comprehensive health care services: a framework for decision-making.* Ottawa: The Association; 1994.

20. Deber R, Lutchmie N, Baranek P, Hilfer N, Duvalko KM, Zlotnik-Shaul R, et al. The public/private mix in health care [commissioned by the National Forum on Health]. In press.

21. Canadian Medical Association. Code of ethics. *CMAJ* 1996;155:1176A-B.

22. Tengs TO, Adams ME, Pliskin JS, Safran DG, Siegel JE, Weinstein MC, et al. Five hundred life-saving interventions and their cost-effectiveness. *Risk Anal* 1995;15:369-90.

23. Mendelssohn DC, Kua BT, Singer PA. Referral for dialysis in Ontario. *Arch Intern Med* 1995;155:2473-8.

24. Olbrisch ME, Levenson JL. Psychosocial evaluation of heart transplant candidates: an international survey of process, criteria and outcomes. *J Heart Lung Transplant* 1991;10:948-55.

25. Levenson JL, Olbrisch ME. Psychosocial evaluation of organ transplant candidates: a comparative survey of process, criteria, and outcome in heart, liver, and kidney transplantation. *Psychosomatics* 1993;34:314-23.

26. Mullen MA, Kohut N, Sam M, Blendis L, Singer PA. Access to adult liver transplantation in Canada: a survey and ethical analysis. *CMAJ* 1996;154:337-42.

27. Jecker NS, Berg AO. Allocating medical resources in rural America: alternative perceptions of justice. *Soc Sci Med* 1992;34:467-74.

28. The Society of Critical Care Medicine Ethics Committee. Attitudes of critical care medicine professionals concerning distribution of intensive care resources. *Crit Care Med* 1994;22:358-62.

29. Zweibel NR, Cassel CK, Karrison T. Public attitudes about the use of chronological age as a criterion for allocating health care resources. *Gerontologist* 1993;33:74-80.

30. Ubel PA, DeKay ML, Baron J, Asch DA. Cost-effectiveness analysis in a setting of budget constraints: Is it equitable? *N Engl J Med* 1996;334:1174-7.

31. Nord E, Richardson J, Kuhse H, Singer P. Maximizing health benefits vs. egalitarianism: an Australian survey of health issues. *Soc Sci Med* 1995;41:1429-37.

32. Baltzan MA. Resource allocation and the Code of Ethics [letter]. *CMAJ* 1998;158(3):298.

Acknowledgement: Drs. Shaf Keshavjee and Michael Fehlings for helpful discussion of the clinical cases.

17

Conflict of interest in research, education and patient care

Trudo Lemmens, Liclur, LLM (Bioethics); Peter A. Singer, MD, MPH

Pharmaflux, a drug manufacturer, invites the director of a residency program, Dr. MM, to attend a 2-hour session on the treatment of unstable angina at a continuing medical education (CME) event in Banff National Park. The session has been organized by Pharmaflux. Dr. MM will receive $3000, and all her expenses will be paid for a 10-day stay. In exchange, she will have to report her impressions of the 2-hour session during a post-conference dinner retreat in Niagara-on-the-Lake, Ont.

Dr. NN did not obtain the federal funding he was counting on for his research project on the efficacy of psychotherapy for the treatment of minor depression. The funding agency to which he applied has experienced significant budget cuts, but Dr. NN hopes that more funding will become available and that he will be successful in the next funding cycle in 6 months' time. He is contacted by a contract research organization to work on a randomized clinical trial comparing the efficacy of a new drug for the treatment of depression with that of standard treatment. If he accepts, he will be able to continue to pay the 2 researchers who have worked with him for the past 4 years. He is asked to sign a confidentiality agreement that would prohibit him from disclosing any results of the study without formal approval by the company. The research firm offers $5000 per patient, to be used at Dr. NN's discretion. Dr. NN calculates that, after deducting administrative costs, compensation for his researchers, and reasonable compensation to the research subjects and himself for the time spent on the study, there will remain $2000 per subject recruited. The research firm suggests that he can use this money for personal expenses.

What is conflict of interest?

A conflict of interest, according to Thompson,[1] "is a set of conditions in which professional judgement concerning a primary interest tends to be unduly influenced by a secondary interest." In the clinical context the primary obligation of physicians is to their patients, whereas in the research context scientific knowledge may be the primary interest. A secondary interest may be of a financial nature, but it may also consist of personal prestige or academic recognition and promotion. In research involving patients, the research interests, although often in concordance with patients' interests, are secondary to clinical care and may conflict with it. To some extent, there may even be a conflict of interest if a person is working as a clinician and a researcher at the same time. A secondary interest may be of an altruistic nature, such as the continued employment of the researchers in the second case described here. A typical example of conflict of interest related to personal gain is physician self-referral.[2] In Thompson's definition the reference to a "set of conditions" is important: having a conflict of interest is an objective situation and does not depend on underlying motives. Therefore, stating that someone has a conflict of interest does not imply a moral condemnation per se. It is the person's actions in the context of a particular situation that may be a cause for concern.

Why is conflict of interest important?

Ethics

Physicians who have conflicts of interest risk damaging the trust between themselves and their patients. Patients rely on physicians' commitment to patient care. They expect that physicians will not be led by motives other than the pursuit of their patients' well-being. If a patient perceives that his or her physician is in a conflict of interest — whether or not the physician is actually influenced by the secondary interest — he or she may lose trust in the physician and in the profession as a whole. Therefore, conflict-of-interest rules safeguard not only the trust of individual patients in their physicians but also the public's trust in the medical profession.

Secondary interests are sometimes so significant that it is only reasonable to predict that some physicians will be influenced by them. Conflict-of-interest rules recognize the inherent danger of some specific situations. In medicine, they are an expression of the principle that, when it comes to patients' well-being, it is better to err on the side of prudence. This means that public interest warrants general preventive measures, not because *most* physicians would act inappropriately in such situations, but because it can be predicted that *some will*.

The imbalance of power between physicians and patients adds to the need for a protective framework. Patients are in a vulnerable position and are dependent on the care of their physicians. This is not an ideal situation from which to judge what weight should be given to the potential impact of secondary interests. Their relatively powerless position makes patients inclined to trust their physicians' decisions. In this context, it seems fair to limit physicians' freedom to engage in activities that could compromise patient care.

It seems impossible to avoid all negative consequences of conflicts of interest. But as Chren and associates indicate,[3] "[p]reserving justice, the trusteeship relationship with our patients, and our own altruism are regulative ideals — that is, standards not always achievable by all of us, but useful templates 'against which all efforts can be measured.'"[3]

Law

The law recognizes that fiduciary duties impose limits on the autonomy and freedom of those in a trusteeship position. A fiduciary relationship is one between unequals in which the more powerful party, such as a physician, is entrusted to protect the best interests or well-being of the less powerful party, such as a patient. In fiduciary relationships, conflict-of-interest rules are notably severe. Citing the Supreme Court case *Hodgkinson* v. *Simms*,[4] Dickens[5] argued that people who are in such positions "are required to act conscientiously to avoid conflict between any of their own interests and those of the dependent party they assume or otherwise come under an obligation to protect" and that courts will hold them "to higher duties of protection of dependent parties' interests."

Conflict-of-interest rules are also integrated into legislation regulating the health care professions. The 1991 Regulated Health Professions Act of Ontario, for example, contains a Health Professions Procedural Code, on the basis of which specific codes for various regulated health care professions have been established. All of these codes prohibit any member of a health care profession from practising the profession "while the member is in a conflict of interest."[6] Many of the codes contain specific examples of professional misconduct, such as charging excessive fees and undertaking unnecessary procedures.

In the 1988 case of *Cox* v. *College of Optometrists of Ontario*[7] the Divisional Court of the Ontario High Court of Justice ruled that professional organizations have the power to impose stringent regulations dealing with conflict of interest. The court defined a conflict of interest as "a personal interest so connected with professional duty that it might reasonably be apprehended to give rise to a danger of actually influencing the exercise of the professional duty."[7] It further ruled that "conflict of interest does not require proof of actual influence by the personal interest upon the professional duty any more than it requires proof of actual receipt of a benefit."[7] The court suggested the following test for determining whether the conflict-of-interest rules of a professional organization are within reasonable boundaries: "Can it be said that no reasonable person could conclude that the prohibited private interest could influence the optometrist's professional conduct?"[7]

Policy

Although there is a traditional body of law on conflict of interest in many other professions, medicine did not start to deal systematically with the issue until the 1980s. Several publications in leading medical journals challenged physicians' participation in the marketing strategies of pharmaceutical companies and expressed concern for some types of interaction between the industry and the medical profession,[3,8,9] and several medical organizations and journals established guidelines on conflict of interest.[9,10] Many medical journals have introduced a requirement that authors disclose any financial interest they have in a study. Some explicitly reject review articles if they are written by people with a financial interest in the review.

In 1990 the American College of Physicians issued a position paper, entitled "Physicians and the pharmaceutical industry," in which it acknowledged that not only real bias but also perceived bias should be avoided.[11] The College recommended, for example, that gifts or subsidies from industry "ought not to be accepted if acceptance might influence or appear to others to influence the objectivity of clinical judgment." More detailed provisions on gifts and conference subsidies can be found in an opinion of the Council on Ethical and Judicial Affairs, which the American Medical Association (AMA) incorporated into its Code of Medical Ethics.[12] Similar restrictions were introduced by the Canadian Medical Association in 1992; its policy on "Physicians and the pharmaceutical industry," updated in 1994, covers a variety of interactions with industry.[13] The policy contains separate sections on research, surveillance studies, CME and clinical evaluation packages. It emphasizes in its "general principles" that "[t]he primary objective of professional interactions between physicians and industry should be the advancement of health of Canadians rather than the private good of either physicians or industry" and that "[r]elationships with the industry are appropriate only insofar as they do not affect the fiduciary nature of the physician–patient relationship." The guidelines do not reject industry sponsorship of research and education but suggest strict rules to maintain an arm's-length relationship between drug manufacturers and physicians. There are many rules, for example, to ensure that CME organizers remain in control of the content of educational events and that any impression of explicit endorsement of a sponsor's product is avoided. When it comes to industry gifts, the CMA guidelines are stricter than those of the AMA. Whereas the AMA allows gifts of "minimal value," the CMA stipulates that "physicians should not accept personal gifts from the pharmaceutical industry." The policy also discourages physicians from investing in drug companies or related undertakings "if knowledge about the success of the company or undertaking might inappropriately affect the manner of their practice or their prescribing behaviour." The policy further states that "the results of any surveillance study will be made available for publication in a peer-reviewed journal within a reasonable period."

In 1993 controversy arose after McMaster University's residency program in internal medicine established more restrictive guidelines, prohibiting lunch briefings by pharmaceutical companies to residents, excluding industry representatives from educational events and rejecting funding when a company insisted on choosing the content of an event.[14] One of the drafters of the guidelines criticized what he perceived as pressure from the industry to soften the guidelines,[15] but others took offence at what they interpreted as a hostile attitude toward industry.[16,17]

The Pharmaceutical Manufacturers Association of Canada has itself established a Code of Marketing Practices, which is similar to the CMA guidelines and explicitly refers to CMA policy, for example, with respect to education events.[18] The weakness of the enforcement mechanism of the code has recently been exposed, and suggestions have been made to improve the current system.[19,20]

Empirical studies

Although perception of harm is an important aspect of conflict of interest, and real harm does not have to be proven, it is interesting to see to what extent physicians interact with industry. Lexchin[21] has provided an excellent overview of the empirical literature between 1978 and 1993. More recently, Hodges[22] reported on interactions between industry and psychiatry residents, interns and clerks, and Sergeant and associates[23] surveyed residents in family medicine. Campbell and colleagues[24] conducted a survey to examine the frequency, importance and potential implications of research-related gifts from companies to academic life scientists and found that 43% of respondents had received a gift independent from a grant or contract. These studies indicate that interactions are omnipresent and range from meetings with pharmaceutical detailers, to attending industry-funded educational events, to receiving gifts and promotional items.

But do these interactions influence physicians and medical researchers? As early as 1982, a study by Avorn and colleagues[8] showed that doctors erroneously believed that their knowledge of 2 popular drugs was based on scientific reports. In reality, their opinion was in line with deceptive advertisements (the published reports indicated that the drugs were not effective for the advertised purposes). Other studies have shown that industry-sponsored education or paid attendance at symposia influences the prescribing patterns of physicians.[21]

Associations have also been shown between the source of funding and the outcome of research studies.[21] One study compared more than 100 clinical trials and found that trials funded by pharmaceutical firms were less likely to conclude that traditional therapy is better than a new drug.[25] Stelfox and collaborators[26] recently reviewed articles on the use of calcium-channel antagonists. They found a strong association between financial relations with the pharmaceutical industry, in particular with producers of calcium-channel antagonists, and support for use of the product. The authors concluded that more effective policies on conflict of interest must be developed.[26] The survey of Campbell and colleagues[24] clearly indicated that most researchers who receive gifts from industry think that industry expects something in return. For example, 32% of recipients reported that the donor expected prepublication review of articles and reports stemming from the use of the gift.[24]

These findings should not come as a surprise. Industry does not reject the concept that interactions have an impact. For example, a publication for the drug market industry suggested that promotional dinners result in an 80% increase in sales of the promoted drug.[27] The clearest indication of the effectiveness of marketing strategies is the amount industry spends on representation and publicity: although the exact amount is a well-kept trade secret, it has been estimated as more than $5 billion in 1992 in the United States[28] and $950 million in Canada.[19]

Surprisingly, many physicians continue to believe that they are not likely to be influenced by their interactions with industry. In one survey of the attitudes of internal medicine faculty and residents, a majority agreed that physicians can be compromised by accepting gifts of high monetary value, but few believed that informational services offered by sales representatives had an influence on their decision-making.[29] Interestingly, Hodges[22] reported that the more money and promotional items residents had received, the more likely they were to believe that these items had not influenced them. Another study, which compared physicians' receipt of gifts, attitudes toward gifts, attitudes toward advertising, influence of interactions with industry on prescription and assessment of prior training, concluded that physicians who received more gifts were not necessarily more positive about the information provided by industry.[30] The authors of that study suggested that physicians are much more discerning than is often thought to be the case. Although the authors concluded that prescribing patterns were not significantly influenced by gifts or other interactions, they did not actually analyse prescribing patterns and physician behaviour. Moreover, patients feel that pharmaceutical gifts are more influential and less appropriate than do their physicians.[31] Overall, most authors and physicians agree that further educational efforts are required to train physicians in their dealings with industry.[22,30]

How should I approach conflict of interest in practice?

There is nothing inherently unethical about interactions between physicians and industry. Private sector support can be highly productive for patients by facilitating research progress and the education of health care providers.

Conflict of interest exists in every aspect of human affairs, including medicine and science. Thus, there is also nothing inherently unethical in finding oneself in a position of conflict of interest. Serious problems arise, however, if one fails to recognize the conflict and address it appropriately.

The first requirement to deal effectively with conflict of interest is awareness. Physicians must realize not only that they may be influenced but also that public perception of influence may harm trust in clinical care and research. Acknowledging conflict of interest is not a confession of moral failure.[32] It is a realistic assessment of the potential impact of secondary interests. Reliance on individual integrity is necessary but not sufficient.[1] Depending on the type of conflict and the potential for real or perceived harm, several strategies are available: disclosure, a system of review and authorization, and prohibition.

Disclosure

Disclosure is the golden rule in conflict of interest. To judge whether one is in a conflict of interest, it can be revealing to ask the question: "Would I feel comfortable if patients and other people found out about my interest in this matter?" If the answer to this question is "no," then disclosure, at a minimum, is prudent. Although trust can be seriously harmed if patients find out about interests that physicians have hidden, trust is likely to be enhanced if patients feel that their physicians are open about it. Colleagues who attend symposia or read articles should be informed of financial ties between presenters and industry. This simply flags that there could be some conscious or unconscious bias in the study result.

The duty to disclose financial interests is recognized in the practice of many medical journals of publishing the financial interests of authors and in the CMA policy, which states that "[t]he physician should be prepared to disclose the nature of such relationships [with industry] to his or her patient, to the organizers and audience of a continuing medical education (CME) event at which he or she is a speaker, and in comparable situations."[13]

Review and authorization

Disclosure of conflicts is one form of external assessment, but laws and regulations have also introduced formal review systems to control conflict of interest, as for example in the context of medical research. Research ethics boards have a mandate to determine, among other things, whether conflicts of interests are affecting the proper conduct of clinical trials and the health care of patients included in the trials. Laws and regulations logically prescribe that members of review boards should themselves not be in a conflict of interest.[33] University policies often include a system of authorization, under which researchers must report financial interests to the university administration. The administration may then verify whether essential conditions (e.g., no restrictions on publications) are met.[34]

Prohibition

Disclosure and review and authorization are not always sufficient. Some conflicts of interest may so deeply affect trust that they ought to be prohibited. The CMA policy disapproves, for example, of researchers who are remunerated over and above reasonable compensation for extra work and loss of other income.[13] Finder's fees, that is, remuneration for merely including research subjects in a clinical trial, ought not to be accepted.[35] In that case, the enticement for including subjects without proper informed consent and without respecting selection criteria is too high. The policy further discourages physicians from accepting a fee from industry in exchange for meetings with representatives or for attending promotional activities.[13] The organizers of CME events are also requested not to "be in a position of conflict of interest by virtue of any relationship" with companies that fund such events.[13]

> Dr. MM has not been invited to make a presentation at the CME event but to report her impressions of the meeting at another leisure event. The prima facie test — "How would people react if I disclose this?" — should suffice to make her reject this proposal. Moreover, the manufacturer is trying to circumvent CMA policy, which provides that "the industry sponsor should not pay for travel or lodging costs or for other personal expenses of physicians attending a CME event."[13] Mere attendance at and reporting on

one session cannot justify this generous offer. Dr. MM should also be wary of the fact that the company organized the session. According to CMA policy, the industry sponsors of an event should not decide on the content and the speakers. Every physician must be aware of the potential for conflict in relationships with industry that are too close, but Dr. MM has reason to be even more prudent. Her decision-making power and her high profile as director of a residency program give her particular duties with respect to ensuring her independence.

Dr. NN's situation represents various levels of conflicting interests. First, scientific interests and industry interests may differ. Dr. NN experiences a conflict because research projects that do not involve drug therapy are of less interest to drug manufacturers. Absence of government funding may inappropriately steer research in only one direction. Although industry-sponsored research is important, public health research and non-drug-related research should also be undertaken. This issue is not within Dr. NN's control, but it is important that he be aware of it and that he continue to strive for a balanced research portfolio. Second, Dr. NN has a legitimate interest in the well-being of his researchers. However, his primary obligations as a physician and a researcher in his own right are toward his patients and toward science. He should only agree to become involved in studies that are of benefit to patients and thus also scientifically valid. Third, as Garfinkel and associates[36] indicate, "[i]t is hard to understand why scholars would become involved in research that is not within their control, especially with regard to the use and publication of data." We would even argue that Dr. NN's obligations as a medical researcher are irreconcilable with the confidentiality agreement he is asked to sign. Even though some form of confidentiality during and shortly after a trial may be appropriate, for example, for patent protection, agreements to that effect should be carefully drafted so that they respect academic freedom and the obligation to protect research subjects from harm. Investigators ought to preserve the right, and even have an obligation, to publish the results of a study.[13] Fourth, Dr. NN should not accept finder's fees for including participants in the trial. This might create conscious or unconscious pressure to be flexible with the inclusion criteria and consent procedures.

References

1. Thompson DF. Understanding financial conflicts of interest. *N Engl J Med* 1993;329:573-6.
2. Cohen L. Issue of fraud raised as MD self-referral comes under spotlight in Ontario. *CMAJ* 1996;154(11):1744-6.
3. Chren MM, Landefeld CS, Murray TH. Doctors, drug companies, and gifts. *JAMA* 1989;262(24):3448-51.
4. *Hodgkinson* v. *Simms* (1994) 117 DLR (4th) 161, 178-9 (C).
5. Dickens B. Conflicts of interest in Canadian health care law. *Am J Law Med* 1995;21:259-80.
6. SO 1991 c 18, cl 51(1)(c).

7. *Cox* v. *College of Optometrists of Ontario* (1988) 65 OR (2d) 461 (Ont Div Ct).
8. Avorn J, Chen M, Hartley R. Scientific versus commercial sources of influence on the prescribing behavior of physicians. *Am J Med* 1982;73:4-8.
9. Relman AS. Dealing with conflicts of interest. *N Engl J Med* 1985;313:749-51.
10. Relman AS. New information for authors and readers. *N Engl J Med* 1990;323:56.
11. American College of Physicians. Physicians and the pharmaceutical industry [position paper]. *Ann Intern Med* 1990;112:624-6.
12. Council on Ethical and Judicial Affairs. Gifts to physicians from the industry (opinion 8.061 of Dec. 3, 1990). *JAMA* 1991;265:501.
13. Canadian Medical Association. Physicians and the pharmaceutical industry (update 1994) [policy summary]. *CMAJ* 1994;150(2):256A-C.
14. Education Council, Residency Training Programme in Internal Medicine, Department of Medicine, McMaster University. Development of residency program guidelines for interaction with the pharmaceutical industry. *CMAJ* 1993;149(4):405-8.
15. Guyatt G. Academic medicine and the pharmaceutical industry: a cautionary tale. *CMAJ* 1994;150(6):951-3.
16. Forrest JB. Faculties of health sciences and the pharmaceutical industry: an effective partnership. *CMAJ* 1994;151(9):1320-2.
17. Arkinstall WW. Interaction between physicians and the pharmaceutical industry [letter]. *CMAJ* 1995;153(4):398-9.
18. Pharmaceutical Manufacturers Association of Canada. *Code of Marketing Practices.* Ottawa: The Association; 1994.
19. Lexchin J. Enforcement of codes governing pharmaceutical promotion: What happens when companies breach advertising guidelines? *CMAJ* 1997;156(3):351-6.
20. Desjardins JG. The PMAC Code of Marketing Practices: Time for improvement? *CMAJ* 1997;156(3):363-4.
21. Lexchin J. Interactions between physicians and the pharmaceutical industry: What does the literature say? *CMAJ* 1993;149(10):1401-7.
22. Hodges B. Interactions with the pharmaceutical industry: experiences and attitudes of psychiatry residents, interns and clerks. *CMAJ* 1995;153(5):553-9.
23. Sergeant MD, Hodgetts G, Godwin M, Walker DMC, McHenry P. Interactions with the pharmaceutical industry: a survey of family medicine residents in Ontario. *CMAJ* 1996;155(9):1243-8.
24. Campbell EG, Louis KS, Blumenthal D. Looking a gift horse in the mouth: corporate gifts supporting life sciences research. *JAMA* 1998;279(13):995-9.
25. Davidson RA. Source of funding and outcome of clinical trials. *J Gen Intern Med* 1986;1:155-8.
26. Stelfox HT, Chua G, O'Rourke K, Detsky AS. Conflict of interest in the debate over calcium-channel antagonists. *N Engl J Med* 1998;338:101-6.
27. Randall T. AMA, Pharmaceutical Association form "solid front" on gift-giving guidelines. *JAMA* 1991;265:2304-5.
28. Pushing drugs to doctors. *Consum Rep* 1992;Feb:87-94.
29. McKinney WP, Schiedermayer DL, Lurie N, Simpson DE, Goodman JL, Rich EC. Attitudes of internal medicine faculty and residents toward professional interaction with pharmaceutical sales representatives. *JAMA* 1990;264(13):1693-7.
30. Aldir RE, Jarjoura D, Phinney M, Poordad F, Guttierez R, Marnejon T, et al. Practicing and resident physicians views on pharmaceutical companies. *J Contin Educ Health Prof* 1996;16:25-31.
31. Gibbons RV, Landry FJ, Blouch DL, Jones DL, Williams FK, Lucey CR, et al. A comparison of physicians and patients attitudes toward pharmaceutical industry gifts. *J Gen Intern Med* 1998;13:151-4.

32. Kassirer JP, Angell M. Financial conflict of interest in biomedical research. *N Engl J Med* 1993;329:570-1.

33. Frances L. IRBs and conflicts of interest. In: Spece RG, Schimm DS, Buchanan AE, editors. *Conflicts of interest in clinical practice and research.* New York: Oxford University Press; 1996. p. 418-36.

34. Bero LA. Disclosure policies for gifts from industry to academic faculty [editorial]. *JAMA* 1998;279:1031-2.

35. Flegel KM. Physicians, finder's fees, and free, informed consent [editorial]. *CMAJ* 1997;157(10):1373-4.

36. Garfinkel PE, Dorian B, Sadavoy J, Bagby RM. Boundary violations and departments of psychiatry. *Can J Psychiatry* 1997;42:764-70.

Acknowledgement: Dr. David Goldbloom for helpful discussions.
Editor's note: In 1998 the CMA updated its 1994 policy on Physicians and The Pharmaceutical Industry. The 1998 policy is available at www.cma.ca/inside/policybase/1998/06-19g.htm

Index

A page number in italic indicates that the information is in a table or figure.